ISGE Series

Series Editor
Andrea R. Genazzani, Endocrinology
International Society of Gynecological Endocrinology
Pisa, Italy

The ISGE Book Series is the expression of the partnership between the International Society of Gynecological Endocrinology and Springer. The book series includes single monographs devoted to gynecological endocrinology relevant topics as well as the contents stemming from educational activities run by ISGRE, the educational branch of the society. This series is meant to be an important tool for physicians who want to advance their understanding of gynecological endocrinology and master this difficult clinical area. The International Society of Gynecological ad Reproductive Endocrinology (ISGRE) School fosters education and clinical application of modern gynecological endocrinology throughout the world by organizing high-level, highly focused residential courses twice a year, the Winter and the Summer Schools. World renowned experts are invited to provide their clinical experience and their scientific update to the scholars, creating a unique environment where science and clinical applications melt to provide the definitive update in this continuously evolving field. Key review papers are published in the Series, thus providing a broad overview over time on the major areas of gynecological endocrinology.

Indexed in Scopus

- **Series Editor: Prof. Andrea R. Genazzani argenazzani@gmail.com and isge.aige@gmail.com**

Andrea R. Genazzani
Angelica Lindén Hirschberg
Alessandro D. Genazzani
Rossella Nappi • Svetlana Vujovic
Editors

Amenorrhea

Volume 10: Frontiers in Gynecological
Endocrinology

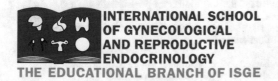

INTERNATIONAL SCHOOL
OF GYNECOLOGICAL
AND REPRODUCTIVE
ENDOCRINOLOGY
THE EDUCATIONAL BRANCH OF ISGE

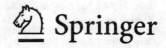

Editors
Andrea R. Genazzani
International Society of Gynecological
Endocrinology
Pisa, Italy

Alessandro D. Genazzani
Department of Obstetrics and Gynecology
University of Modena and Reggio Emilia
MODENA, Modena, Italy

Svetlana Vujovic
Faculty of Medicine
Clinic of Endocrinology
Diabetes and Diseases of Metabolism
University of Belgrade
University Clinical Center of Serbia
Belgrade, Serbia

Angelica Lindén Hirschberg
Department of Gynecology and
Reproductive Medicine
Karolinska University Hospital
Stockholm, Sweden

Rossella Nappi
Research Center for Reproductive
Medicine, Gynecological Endocrinology
and Menopause
IRCCS San Matteo Foundation
Pavia, Italy

ISSN 2197-8735   ISSN 2197-8743   (electronic)
ISGE Series

ISBN 978-3-031-22380-8   ISBN 978-3-031-22378-5   (eBook)
https://doi.org/10.1007/978-3-031-22378-5

This Springer imprint is published by the registered company Springer Nature Switzerland AG
The registered company address is: Gewerbestrasse 11, 6330 Cham, Switzerland

Contents

Müllerian Malformations and Their Treatments

Efthymios Deligeoroglou and Vasileios Karountzos

Abbreviation

MM   Müllerian malformations

1.1   Introduction

Müllerian malformations (MM) are the anomalies resulting from failure of fusion of the paramesonephric ducts in the middle line, during their connection with the urogenital sinus. They occur due to alterations in the formation of the upper vaginal lumen and the uterine lumen, and also because of non-absorption of the septum in the fusion of ducts. Their clinical expression varies from very light disorders to serious obstetrical conditions such as vaginal and uterine agenesis, which is called the Mayer-Rokitansky-Küster-Hauser (MRKH) syndrome [1]. The prevalence of congenital uterine anomalies according to Saravelos et al. [2] was found to be 6.7% in general population, 7.3% in sterile women, and 16.7% in women who had recurrent miscarriages. The septate uterus seems to be the most common anomaly in infertile women and the arcuate uterus the most common among those who have habitual abortion. In another study, Nahum [3] found the above mentioned statistics to be 0.5%, 0.17%, and 3.5%, respectively. What is of great importance is that müllerian

E. Deligeoroglou (✉)
Medical School, National and Kapodistrian University of Athens, Athens, Greece

Division of Pediatric-Adolescent Gynecology, MITERA Children's Hospital, Athens, Greece

V. Karountzos
Division of Pediatric-Adolescent Gynecology, MITERA Children's Hospital, Athens, Greece

© International Society of Gynecological Endocrinology 2023
A. R. Genazzani et al. (eds.), *Amenorrhea*, ISGE Series,
https://doi.org/10.1007/978-3-031-22378-5_1

anomalies present with great diversity giving many diagnostic and treatment options and doubts, while most of the studies include isolated cases or small case series focusing on the obstruction of menstrual flow, obstetric complications, and/or history of sterility [4].

1.2 Prevalence

The prevalence of congenital uterine anomalies in unselected populations is 5.5%, while in infertile patients is 8.0%. This prevalence, especially in infertile women, is not increased and it is approximately the same as that in fertile patients with normal reproductive outcomes [5]. When infertile and fertile women were included in the same study, septate uterus was found in 35%, bicornuate in 26%, arcuate in 18%, unicornuate in 10%, didelphys in 8%, while aplasia in 3% [5]. It is well understood that these frequencies vary regarding the populations that are studied, as well as the criteria that are used to identify these abnormalities. In another well-designed study, including patients with normal reproductive outcomes, septate uterus was found in 90%, bicornuate in 5%, while didelphys in 5% [6].

1.3 Etiopathology

Sexual differentiation is a continuous process that starts with the fertilization of the ovule by the sperm. In women, the normal absence of müllerian inhibitory factor results in degeneration of the mesonephric ducts to paramesonephric ducts. These structures, which are bilateral, suffer from stretching in around the ninth week of pregnancy and remain open and separated in the upper segment, thus originating in the fallopian tubes. In the lower segment, they form after their junction in the upper 2/3 of the vagina [1]. As the fusion has been completed, the septum between the paramesonephric ducts starts to be absorbed and finally the uterovaginal canal. Uterus has a normal shape around the 12th week of pregnancy and is totally completed in the 22nd week [7]. The development of the vagina depends on the fusion between the urogenital sinus with the müllerian structures. Therefore, the upper 4/5 of the vagina is of müllerian origin and the lower 1/5 has its origin in the urogenital sinus. The epithelium of the upper 1/3 of the vagina originates in the uterovaginal primordium and the lower 2/3 in the urogenital sinus, and the hymen is a sign of the endodermal membrane [8]. What is independent of this process is the ovaries, which are developed from cells of a different origin, and as a result they are not associated with müllerian anomalies [1, 9]. Due to the same mesodermal origin of the genital and urinary tracts, any paramesonephric anomaly could be associated with renal anomaly, which should always be investigated in these patients. Congenital malformation of female genital tracts is a result of a failure during embryogenesis, and the most common genes taking part in this procedure are HOXA13 (hand-foot-genital syndrome) [10] and HOXA10, expressed in the embryonic paramesonephric ducts [11]. Genital anomalies induced by environmental agents such as diethylstilbestrol and thalidomide are also described in the literature. It is of great importance that the type of malformation depends on the moment that the failure occurs, and the earlier in pregnancy it takes place, the more serious the malformation is. Therefore, complete aplasia associated with urinary malfunctions may be seen if the pathology occurs between the 6th and 9th weeks of pregnancy, and on the other hand total or partial septation, rarely associated with urinary malformations, may be observed if the problem occurs between the 13th and 17th weeks of pregnancy.

1.4   Classification Systems

Starting from the nineteenth century, several classifications have been proposed based on embryology and development of müllerian ducts, but these classification systems have several difficulties not only in terminologies, but also in failure in the characterization of the anomalies. The goal was the same, in all cases, to make the diagnosis more accurate, as well as to help distinguish cases, but the problem remained with no consensus in relation to their use. Among those, the classification VCUAM (Vagina Cervix Uterus Adnex-associated Malformation) [12] can be cited as well as that proposed by Acien and Acien [6]. Currently, the most used is the one proposed by Buttram and Gibbons [13], accepted and modified in 1988 by the American Fertility Society (AFS), today the American Society of Reproductive Medicine (ASRM) [14], which separates the anomalies into seven classes (Fig. 1.1). The European Society of Human Reproduction and Embryology (ESHRE) and the European Society for Gynaecological Endoscopy (ESGE) [14] developed another

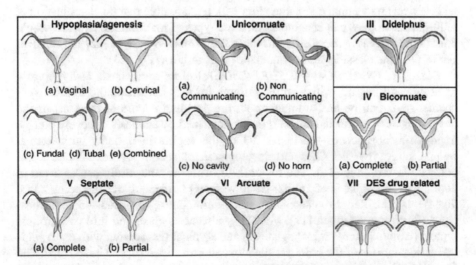

Fig. 1.1 The AFS/ASRM class ification system. Adapted by the American Fertility Society. The American Fertility Society classification of adnexal adhesions, distal tubal occlusion secondary or tubal ligation, tubal pregnancies, müllerian anomalies, and intrauterine adhesions. Fertil Steril 1988;49(6):944–55

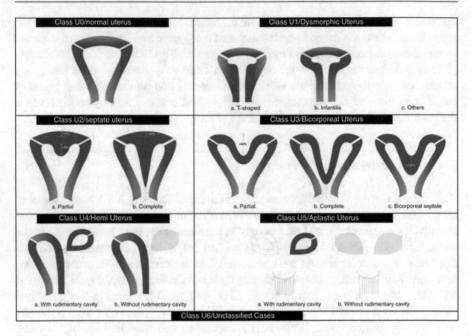

Fig. 1.2 The ESGE/ESHRE classification system. Adapted by Grimbizis GF, Di Spiezio Sardo A, Saravelos SH, Gordts S, Exacoustos C, Van Schoubroeck D, et al. The Thessaloniki ESHRE/ESGE consensus on diagnosis of female genital anomalies. Hum Reprod 2016;31(1):2–7

classification based on anatomy, embryological origin, degree of uterine deformity, and cervical and vaginal anomalies (Fig. 1.2). It is possible that no classification of müllerian anomalies can encompass all these types of malformations, which could present themselves in many different ways. Based on AFS-ASRM [12] and ESHRE/ESGE [14], the classification of anomalies is as follows (Fig. 1.3):

Class 1 (AFS)/U5bC4V4 (ESHRE/ESGE): Refers to agenesis or hypoplasia of uterus and vagina, which in its extreme form is known as the MRKH syndrome. As it can be easily understood, the problem occurs at the start of the development of müllerian ducts. It is characterized by agenesis or severe uterine hypoplasia, absence of the upper 2/3 of the vagina in patients with normal female karyotype (46,XX), and development of secondary sexual characters compatible with age [15]. The lower third of the vagina rarely passes 2 cm in depth. Its prevalence is of 1/4500–5000 women [1, 16] and, despite being a rare disease, is considered the second most common cause of primary amenorrhea, right after hypogonadism [17]. MRKH syndrome is classified into two groups: typical (isolated uterovaginal agenesis) and atypical (associated with extra genital malformations of the kidneys, skeleton, auditory system, and heart) [15]. The first clinical experience of these patients is primary amenorrhea and incapacity for vaginal coitus, while renal malformations are the commonest concomitant lesions, varying from 15 to 34%.

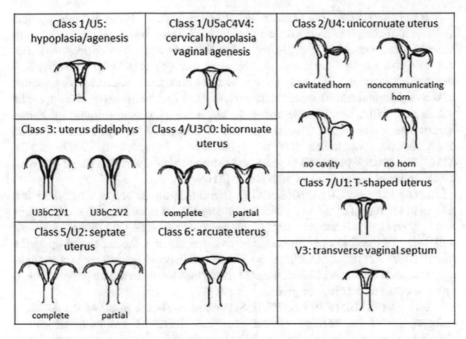

Fig. 1.3 The combination of ESHRE/ESGE and AFS/ASRM system. Adapted by Ludwin A, Ludwin I. Comparison of the ESHRE-ESGE and ASRM classifications of müllerian duct anomalies in everyday practice. Hum Reprod 2015; 30:569–80

Class 1/U5aC4V4 (ESHRE/ESGE): Congenital cervical atresia occurs in 1/80,000–1,000,000 women [18]. Most of the times, it is associated with total or partial aplasia of the vagina and renal anomalies. Not rarely, a hematometra is observed due to the menstrual blood that has no way to flow out, while the fallopian tubes can be distended leading in some cases to an acute hemorrhagic abdomen. It should be diagnosed and treated immediately due to its significant morbidity and mortality.

Class 2 (AFS)/U4 (ESHRE/ESGE): The unicornuate uterus is the result of inability of one of the müllerian ducts to migrate to its correct place; therefore, a failure in the unilateral development occurs. This uterine horn can be unique, when there is complete agenesis of one of the müllerian ducts (U4b), or accompanied by another rudimentary uterine horn, which could be of three types: without cavity (U4b), cavitated, or cavitated noncommunicating horn (U4a). What is of great importance is that the endometrium in the latter corn undergoes hormonal stimulation and its cavity progressively increases in volume due to the retention of menstrual blood, which has no way of flowing out. This causes pain many times of cyclic origin, leading to an increased volume in abdomen. These women unfortunately may have obstetrical complications such as miscarriages, restriction of intrauterine growth, and premature birth labor. Unicornuate uterus represents 0.3–4% of the uterine anomalies and occurs in 1/5400 women, while 74–90% are associated with rudimentary horn [19, 20].

Class 3 (AFS)/U3bC2V1 or U3bC2V2 (ESHRE/ESGE): Uterus didelphys occurs as a result of complete failure of fusion of both müllerian ducts. However, development of uterus continues individually, giving rise to two uterine cavities, two cervices, and two vaginas separated, and between them there will be a longitudinal septum, while menstrual flow is normal. In rare cases, the septum can obstruct one of the vaginas and cause menstrual flow retention of that hemi-uterus causing cyclic pelvic pain, with a result of hematocolpos, hematometra, hematosalpinx, and hematoperitoneum. If ipsilateral renal agenesis is observed, the syndrome is called Herlyn-Werner-Wunderlich (HWW) syndrome and represents 3–4% of the MM. The obstetric prognosis is good, and there are also reported cases of pregnancies with twins with a fetus in each uterus [21].

Class 4 (AFS)/U3C0 (ESHRE/ESGE): Bicornuate uterus occurs when there is a failure in the fusion of the two müllerian structures that results in two uterine horns and only one cervix. Complete or partial bicornuate uterus depends on the degree of deficiency of the fusion, so in complete case the cavities are separated up to the internal orifice of the cervix and are not linked and in partial case there is some linkage. It represents around 10% of the MM, is asymptomatic in the majority of cases, and can cause miscarriage or premature birth [22].

Class 5 (AFS)/U2 (ESHRE/ESGE): Septate uterus is the result of the deficit in reabsorption of the median septum after the fusion of müllerian structures. Depending on the moment when the failure occurs, the septum can be complete or partial and the external contour of the uterus is always normal. The structure of the septum can be muscular or fibrous, and this diagnostic is extremely important for therapeutic approach. It represents 55% of the malformations and is associated with recurrent miscarriage and premature birth. It is one of the malformations with the worst results in relation to reproduction [22, 23].

Class 6 (AFS): Arcuate uterus is also considered a variant of the normal with no clinical translation [12]. Eventually, it can be the cause of reproductive alteration when no other problem is detected. It occurs due to the failure in the final stage of reabsorption of the intermüllerian septum and does not need intervention.

Class 7 (AFS)/U1 (ESHRE/ESGE): This is induced by diethylstilbestrol, represented by a T-shaped uterus detected in daughters of women who used this drug during pregnancy. The uterine cavity is irregular and hypoplastic; there are poor chances for pregnancy and high risk of miscarriage or ectopic pregnancy [24]. Diethylstilbestrol was discontinued in 1971, and, for this reason, this is an increasingly rare anomaly, which tends to disappear.

V3 (ESHRE/ESGE): Transverse vaginal septum results from the failure of canalization of the vaginal plaque at the point where the urogenital sinus meets the müllerian duct, and it is not associated with other malformations. Women with a perforated septum take more time to have a diagnosis because they menstruate normally and there are few symptoms. The thickness and localization are extremely important to define the treatment: the lowest, the thinnest, and the perforated ones have better results, while the highest and the thickest ones have great chances of complications such as rectovaginal fistula and hysterectomy. Its occurrence is estimated to be between 1/2100 and 1/72,000 women [25].

1.5   Clinical Manifestations

Primary amenorrhea which is defined as the absence of menses at age 15, in the presence of normal growth and secondary sexual characteristics, is one of the commonest clinical expression of congenital uterine anomalies, especially in uterine and vaginal aplasia, while another common symptom is cyclic pelvic pain, in which a possible outflow tract obstruction should be evaluated or prolonged or otherwise there will be abnormal bleeding at the time of menarche, recurrent pregnancy loss, or preterm delivery, and thus may be identified in patients, including adolescents, who present with these disorders. Moreover, a longitudinal vaginal septum may be found in clinical examination, while others may be detected when imaging studies are performed to evaluate patients with infertility, symptoms related to nonreproductive organ systems, or trauma. As mentioned above, patients with congenital uterine anomalies are at increased risk of having renal, skeletal, or abdominal wall abnormalities, or a history of inguinal hernia, and vice versa. The most common renal anomalies are duplex collecting system, horseshoe kidney, pelvic kidney, and unilateral renal agenesis and are most commonly associated with an obstructed hemiuterus, obstructed hemivagina, and transverse vaginal septa.

Even though MM, in most cases, do not prevent conception and implantation, obstetric complications such as spontaneous abortion, recurrent miscarriage, fetal growth restriction, preterm delivery, antepartum and postpartum bleeding, placental attachment abnormalities, cervical insufficiency, fetal malpresentation, pregnancy-associated hypertension, increased possibility of cesarean delivery, and rarely rupture of a rudimentary horn may be observed [12, 17–25]. Some clinical expressions such as malpresentation and increased possibility of cesarean delivery can be explained easily by the small uterine cavity of the anomalous uterus, which may inhibit fetal movement to cephalic presentation [26], while growth restriction may be related to abnormal uterine vasculature. Postpartum hemorrhage may result from an abnormal attachment of placenta, while pregnancy-associated hypertension has been attributed to coexistent congenital renal abnormalities [22] and pregnancy loss may be related to implantation at an unfavorable site, especially in the presence of a septum [12]. Many patients are asymptomatic, and findings are first presented in a routine physical examination which leads to further evaluation and diagnosis.

1.6   Diagnostic Methods

Clinical examination is playing a crucial role in MM. In cases of primary amenorrhea, clinical examination should be focused on the presence of secondary sexual characteristics as well as on the presence or absence of the uterus. Blood tests focused on follicle-stimulating hormone (FSH) levels may be very helpful. If FSH is normal and clinical examination—ultrasound—indicates that the uterus is absent, the probable diagnosis is müllerian agenesis or androgen insensitivity syndrome. In the case of müllerian agenesis, the circulating testosterone is in the normal range for women, and in the case of androgen insensitivity, the circulating testosterone is in the male range and testes may be present in the inguinal area or found intra-abdominal on ultrasound. Karyotype is always helpful in these cases because in agenesis karyotype is normal female 46,XX, in contrast to androgen insensitivity syndrome which is 46,XY. In addition, the vagina and cervix should be examined for anatomic abnormalities. Anatomic abnormalities that can cause primary amenorrhea include an intact hymen, transverse vaginal septum, or vaginal agenesis, also known as müllerian agenesis or Mayer-Rokitansky-Küster-Hauser (MRKH) syndrome [4]. A careful genital examination should be performed for clitoral size, pubic hair development, intactness of the hymen, and vaginal length. If the vagina cannot be penetrated with a small cotton swab (Q-tip) or finger, rectal examination may allow evaluation of the internal organs.

Over the past years, imaging diagnostic tools have been constantly improving. The initial diagnostic method is the two-dimensional ultrasound (US2D), but also used are three-dimensional ultrasound (US3D), MRI, hysterosalpingo-contrast sonography, X-ray hysterosalpingography, video hysteroscopy, and video laparoscopy.

US2D is the initial method because it is simple, noninvasive, low cost, and usually available and provides good information; however, it is highly dependent on the experience of the examiner [26–28]. US3D has good reproducibility and high level of agreement among different observers, provides additional and more reliable images, and allows for the evaluation of the cervix and the vagina; however, it is less available and requires more specialized training than the US2D [26–29].

MRI is considered the gold standard method and offers objective and reliable tridimensional information about all aspects of anatomy, except for the tubes; it can be used in all cases, including obstructive malformations. It is more expensive and less available than the US and needs a qualified professional to interpret the results [26, 30–32]. MRI is also very helpful in girls who develop endometriosis from retrograde menstruation from obstructed uterine horns.

Hysterosalpingo-contrast sonography is a minimally invasive and low-cost method and provides good information about the cervix and uterine cavity but is highly dependent on the examiner, and the distention of the uterine cavity can modify its internal contours generating false-negative images [26, 33]. X-ray hysterosalpingography provides information only about the uterine cavity and tubes and is used more in cases of infertility. It is an invasive, painful exam and does not evaluate the external contour, does not differentiate the septate uterus from the bicornuate one, does not diagnose the noncommunicating uterine horn, and cannot be used in vaginal and cervical obstructions [26, 34].

Hysteroscopy is minimally invasive and provides reliable information about the vagina, cervical canal, and uterine cavity, although it does not evaluate the external contours or the thickness of the uterine wall and does not differentiate the septate uterus from the bicornuate one [26]. Laparoscopy evaluates the external contour of the uterus and the peritoneal structures, but it is an invasive exam, does not evaluate the thickness of the uterine wall, and completely depends on the experience and subjective evaluation of the examiner [26]. When obstructed uterine horns with the presence of active endometrium without an associated cervix and upper vagina are identified, then laparoscopic removal of the unilateral or bilateral obstructed uterine structures should be performed [35]. In most cases, surgical excision of the uterine horn results in improvement of the endometriosis [5].

Multiple studies have confirmed the prevalence of renal anomalies in patients with müllerian agenesis to be 27–29%; therefore, ultrasound evaluation of the kidneys is warranted for all patients [36, 37]. Skeletal anomalies (e.g., scoliosis, vertebral arch disturbances, hypoplasia of the wrist) have been reported in approximately 8–32% of patients; therefore, spine radiography (X-ray) may reveal a skeletal anomaly even in asymptomatic patients [36–38].

1.7 Treatment

1.7.1 Which Classification Is Better for Patient Management?

According to the authors of the ESHRE/ESGE system, their classification contains a clear definition of all types of anomaly, and the anomalies are categorized in well-described classes and subclasses as mentioned above, and the ESHRE/ESGE criteria allow objective classification of uterine morphology [26]. However, other studies have shown that the ESHRE/ESGE classification system for main classes has significant methodologic issues [39, 40]. Importantly, three groups of researchers have highlighted that the ESHRE/ESGE system can lead to unnecessary surgical procedures for conditions that appear to be benign uterine variants [40–42]. Moreover, the ESHRE/ESGE system and their criteria included updated definitions and were not created for patient management as authors stated [14, 26]. A recent systematic review indicates that current evidence favors continued use of the ASRM classification [43]. In conclusion, it is still very difficult to answer the question of which system is better, because all systems have potential advantages and disadvantages. All systems are arbitrary, with overlapping features.

1.7.2 Congenital Uterine Malformations by Experts (CUME): Definitions 2018

The use of different criteria and definitions, especially in Europe and the United States, as well as different local classifications is a significant barrier for communication between practitioners, experts, and researchers. What would be a good idea is the creation of a single global classification system using the most voted options of independent international top experts as reference to find a common language for classification of anomalies. Recently, the Congenital Uterine Malformations by Experts (CUME) group was created for that reason and is the first definition, which is available in order to reflect the diagnosis made most often by experts for distinguishing normal/arcuate and septate uterus [44].

Furthermore, surgical approaches to treating MM are always evolving. Advances in imaging have allowed for noninvasive and more accurate diagnosis of anomalies, which has resulted in better surgical planning with fewer diagnostic surgeries needed. Technologic advances in surgical equipment, as well as laparoscopy, have helped in better correction of these anomalies. In addition, past surgical approaches with the focus on correction of MM for patient's symptom relief, without any consideration for future fertility, are not nowadays in the surgical plan and most experts allow individuals to take part in their future reproductive option, which is well discussed most of the times with their parents.

Moreover, minimally invasive techniques have today replaced all past surgical approaches. The most significant impact has been with the hysteroscopic incision of uterine septum, which replaced the Jones [45] or Tompkins [46] metroplasty performed at laparotomy [47]. The hysteroscopic septum incision can be done as a same-day surgery, with significantly shorter recovery and less pain, and importantly allows the young girl to have a vaginal delivery without a significant risk of uterine rupture [8]. In some cases, hysteroscopic septum incision is performed under laparoscopic control, in order to prevent excessive incision and fundal perforation. Currently, ultrasound guidance, later performed abdominally [48], has replaced more invasive laparoscopy [40]. Resection of the septum hysteroscopically can improve pregnancy outcome [49]. Other examples for past procedures that now have been replaced by others in order to preserve the reproductive function include hysterectomy for treatment of a patient with a high transverse vaginal septum or cervical agenesis, hemi-hysterectomy with vaginectomy for obstructed hemiuterus in blind hemivagina, and amputative or ablative surgery of blind obstructed hemicavity in Robert septate uterus [50].

In case of uterus didelphys, 20% of patients also have unilateral anomalies, such as an obstructed hemivagina and ipsilateral renal agenesis. In addition, there may be a microcommunication between the patent vagina and the obstructed vagina, resulting in an infected obstructed hemivagina, while bilateral complete obstruction is also possible and presents with primary amenorrhea. Treatment involves resection of the wall of the obstructed vagina followed by creation of a single vaginal vault.

Metroplasty should be considered for patients with pelvic pain, recurrent miscarriages, or a history of preterm delivery. Today's data do not support the fact that abdominal repair of the didelphic uterus improves pregnancy outcomes. In the unicornuate uterus, care should be taken to assess for the presence of a noncommunicating or rudimentary horn. Even though most rudimentary horns are asymptomatic, some contain functional, but not necessarily normal [51], endometrium that is shed cyclically. But if a rudimentary horn is obstructed (without communication to the other uterus or cervix), as mentioned above, the patient may develop cyclic or chronic abdominopelvic pain and may require surgical excision of the obstructed horn [51].

Bicornuate uterus is not a cause of difficulty conceiving, but rather a recurrent miscarriage in the second trimester of pregnancy and premature birth. When no other cause is identified, Strassman's metroplasty can be recommended, with good results and a 90% rate of full pregnancy [52]. Transverse vaginal septum should be treated with surgical resection and anastomosis of the proximal and distal vaginas. The choice of the technique depends on its localization and thickness, which is diagnosed in a physical exam, US, and MRI, and it can be vaginal or laparoscopic. The lowest, the thinnest, and the perforated ones have the best results, and the main complications are stenosis, re-obstruction, dyspareunia, and psychological difficulties. Vaginal dilatation is generally recommended after surgery to improve the result [53].

In case of MRKH syndrome, primary vaginal elongation by dilation is the appropriate first-line approach in most patients because it is safer, patient controlled, and more cost effective than surgery. Vaginal dilation is successful for more than 90–96% of patients; therefore, surgery should be reserved for the rare patient who is unsuccessful with primary dilator therapy or who prefers surgery after a thorough informed consent discussion with her gynecologic care provider and her respective parent(s). Regardless of the surgical technique chosen, referrals to centers with expertise should be offered and the surgeon must be experienced with the procedure. The primary aim of surgery is the creation of a vaginal canal to allow penetrative intercourse. The timing of the surgery depends on the patient and the type of procedure planned. Surgical procedures often are performed in late adolescence or young adulthood when the patient is mature enough to agree to the procedure and to be able to adhere to postoperative dilation. Common complications in vaginoplasty include bladder or rectal perforation, graft necrosis, hair-bearing vaginal skin, and fistulae [54].

Several techniques have been used for vaginoplasty, and there is not a worldwide consensus for the best, in order to afford the best functional outcome and sexual satisfaction [55]. Historically, the most common surgical procedure used to create a neovagina has been the modified Abbe–McIndoe operation. This procedure involves the dissection of a space between the rectum and bladder, placement of a stent covered with a split-thickness skin graft into the space, and diligent use of vaginal dilation postoperatively. Other procedures for the creation of neovagina are the Vecchietti procedure and other laparoscopic modifications of operations previously performed by laparotomy [56]. The laparoscopic Vecchietti procedure is a modification of the open technique in which a neovagina is created using an external traction device that is affixed temporarily to the abdominal wall [57]. Another procedure, the Davydov procedure, was developed as a three-stage operation that requires dissection of the rectovesicular space with abdominal mobilization of a segment of the peritoneum and subsequent attachment of the peritoneum to the introitus [58–61]. Other vaginoplasty graft options include bowel, buccal mucosa, amnion and various other allografts. Last but not least, Williams vaginoplasty is a very reliable and worldwide used method of vaginoplasty. The Creatsas modification of Williams vaginoplasty is a fast and simple technique, in which a perineal skin flap is used to create a perineal pouch. During this procedure, the tissues of the perineum are mobilized and the inner skin margins of the created flap are stitched together using absorbable sutures. Regarding this technique, we have a large series of neovagina creation, with more than 247 adolescents, with no past surgical complications and perfect sexual life as reported by women later in their life.

Another issue in MRKH syndrome is uterine transplantation. This is an innovative approach to treat fertility due to MM [62]. Procurement of the donor uterus has traditionally been performed at laparotomy from a living or deceased donor. Traditionally, uterus harvest for a live transplant involves a long and complicated procedure to remove the uterus and its vascular supply without causing undue trauma to the donor. Recently, the first case report of robotic assisted laparoscopic harvesting was described for procurement of a uterus from a live donor [63]. The donor undergoes a procedure similar to a radical hysterectomy, with removal of the ovaries to obtain adequate ovarian vascular pedicles, both arterial and venous, to allow perfusion of the uterus in the recipient. As the robotic assisted laparoscopic approach has become common place for performing a radical hysterectomy, it is natural that this approach may be used for the uterus donor and allows for a quicker recovery.

1.8 Controversies

1.8.1 Uterovaginal Anastomosis for Cervical Agenesis

As surgical approaches evolve to take into consideration reproductive choices and patient input, controversies in management have developed. Management of cervical agenesis has traditionally involved performing a hysterectomy primarily to treat the pain caused by hematometra and sequelae of retrograde menstruation, including endometriosis, hematosalpinx, and hematoperitoneum. Some case series evaluating outcomes of uterovaginal fistula showed poor outcomes. The frequency of reoperation and hysterectomy of girls undergoing uterovaginal reconstruction for cervical agenesis ranged from 10 to >50%, while sepsis is always an issue in these cases and sometimes is fatal [64–67]. Pregnancies reported after uterovaginal anastomosis are few [65, 66], due to the high incidence of tubal damage and adhesive disease from retrograde menstruation. On the other hand, surgical approaches are evolving; therefore, in one study of 18 cases, all of the women had successful reconstruction and only one woman experienced restenosis, which was treated successfully with the use of canalization [68]. Pregnancy occurred without assistance in ten women, and four women had a successful delivery via cesarean section at 36–38 weeks. Another case series of laparoscopic assisted uterovaginal anastomosis involved 14 patients, with 9 undergoing concomitant vaginoplasty [69]. Only one patient underwent hysterectomy, owing to restenosis and infection. Unassisted pregnancy was achieved in three of five patients who were sexually active. The better outcomes in these studies have brought into question which management is appropriate. Although hysterectomy is a "safer" option because it avoids potential complications of restenosis, infection, and death, it does not allow for the individual to preserve her uterus for cultural or emotional reasons or to carry a pregnancy.

1.8.2 Surgery of Septate Uterus by Different Definitions

Septate uterus as a definition is under controversies through all these years, while an issue always arises according to whether or not surgical treatment improves clinical outcomes. As discussed above, the ASRM and ESHRE/ESGE classification systems differ in the diagnosis of septate uterus [44]. The median internal indentation in those diagnosed as septate according to the ESHRE/ESGE criteria was 10.7 mm (lower-upper quartile 8.1–20 mm), whereas for those diagnosed as septate according to the ASRM criteria, the median indentation was 21.1 mm (lower-upper quartile 18.8–33.1 mm); therefore, in ESHRE/ESGE system, septate uterus is overdiagnosed [26]. Currently, randomized trials are underway to evaluate outcomes following uterine septum treatment versus expectant management [42, 70]. However, more studies are needed to determine if surgical correction of a uterine septum defined by ESHRE/ ESGE, ASRM, or other criteria improves clinical outcomes.

1.8.3 Cervical Septum Preservation and Resection

Treatment of complete septate uterus by hysteroscopy may involve preservation of the cervical septum or resection. One randomized study compared surgical treatment of uterine septum with and without cervical septum resection in 28 patients [71]. In the group who had preservation of the cervical septum, operating times were longer, incidence of bleeding >150 mL higher, and cesarean section rate higher than in the group who underwent cervical septum incision. There were no differences in reproductive outcomes between the two groups. However, another case series reported need for cerclage in 5 out of 22 patients owing to cervical shortening when cervical septum was removed [72]. Commonly, interstitial cases of the septate and double cervix (wide septa or septate/double cervix) are present, and the strict distinction between these two conditions may be a challenge and even impossible.

1.8.4 Blind Hemivagina

Double uterus with obstructed hemivagina is a well-recognized müllerian anomaly [73]. This anomaly is also known as obstructed hemivagina with renal anomaly and as Herlyn-Werner-Wunderlich syndrome [74, 75]. This obstructed hemivagina is seen primarily in association with uterus didelphys or complete septate uterus, and sometimes with bicornuate uterus with double uterine cavity and cervical canal. Many treatment options have been proposed. Treatment most commonly has been a vaginal approach to resect the vaginal septum, relieve the obstruction, and allow a single common vaginal canal. However, hysteroscopic resection has also been used to resect vaginal septum in a virginal patient when preservation of the hymen is desired [72–75].

1.9 Challenges and Ongoing and Further Studies

It is well understood that all these years, many steps forward have been made regarding diagnosis, classification, and management of MM. However, many questions remain unanswered and need further evaluation and studies. Good-quality studies on prevalence and clinical implications, with measurable criteria, are required for distinguishing what are normal and abnormal conditions. Studies focused on obvious morphologies, such as normal/arcuate, septate, bicornuate, and didelphys uterus, and other debatable conditions, such as T-shaped uterus, with the use of measurable criteria for diagnosis should be performed. Surgical interventions in women with infertility and recurrent pregnancy loss who have potentially benign morphologic variants of uterus can show good reproductive outcome after correction. But it is not sufficient evidence to conclude that surgery is truly helpful for these women. Currently, there are two ongoing randomized controlled trials focused on septate uterus. As mentioned above, the protocols raise questions about the validity of the definitions of septate uterus used. On the other hand, performing randomized controlled trials in women with unique anomalies is not easy and sometimes impossible. One of the best ideas may be creation of an international registry of anomalies and comparison of reproductive outcomes depending on the approaches. Such a registry should include datasets from accurate diagnostic methods, such as 3D ultrasound and MRI that can be reliably reanalyzed [76–78].

1.10   Discussion

The various MM present themselves in diverse forms and in different phases of a woman's life. The two principal classifications used currently, that of AFS-ASRM and of ESHRE/ESGE, encompass the majority of cases, although there are others and there is still not a consensus. There are isolated cases of MM that do not fit into any of the classifications. Women with more impacting symptoms such as primary amenorrhea, incapacity for vaginal coitus, or pelvic pain, due to obstruction of the menstrual flow, are diagnosed earlier because they seek assistance earlier. However, those women experiencing problems related to reproduction, such as recurrent pregnancy loss, premature birth, and infertility, many times only have diagnosis of genital malformation during the investigation of these symptoms. Clinical examination has a major role in diagnosis, although US2D is the first imaging exam used, followed by MRI, which for some authors is the gold standard imaging exam. The clinical presentation and treatment for MM are directly related to the anatomy of the defect. Malformations that obstruct the menstrual flow should be treated rapidly doing a suitable surgical procedure for each case. Patients with vaginal agenesis may undergo vaginoplasty or vaginal dilatation through diverse techniques. Due to the frequent association between MM and urinary anomalies, the finding of any of the types should lead to the investigation of the other. Since it is a rare pathology, the majority of studies found in the literature are composed of case reports, small series of cases, and comparative studies and many authors just report the experience of their service. Studies involving genetics and embryology, as well as randomized studies, are necessary, so that one can understand and treat, in an increasingly better fashion, women who are born having to deal with the fact that they are different.

Acknowledgements Nothing to declare.

Conflict of Interest Nothing to declare.

References

1. Pizzo A, Lagana AS, Sturlese E, Retto G, Retto A, De Dominici R, et al. Mayer-Rokitansky-Kuster-Hauser syndrome: embryology, genetics and clinical and surgical treatment. ISRN Obstet Gynecol. 2013;2013:628–717.
2. Saravelos SH, Cocksedge KA, Li TC. Prevalence and diagnosis of congenital uterine anomalies in women with reproductive failure: a critical appraisal. Hum Reprod Update. 2008;14(5):415–29.
3. Nahum GG. Uterine anomalies. How common are they, and what is their distribution among subtypes? J Reprod Med. 1998;43(10):877–87.
4. Jones HW Jr. Reproductive impairment and the malformed uterus. Fertil Steril. 1981;36(2):137–48.
5. American Fertility Society. The American Fertility Society classification of adnexal adhesions, distal tubal occlusion secondary or tubal ligation, tubal pregnancies, mullerian anomalies and intrauterine adhesions. Fertil Steril. 1988;49(6):944–55.
6. Acien P, Acien MI. The history of female genital tract malformation: classification and proposal of an updated system. Hum Reprod Update. 2011;17:693–705.
7. Jost A. A new look at the mechanism controlling sex differentiation in mammals. Johns Hopkins Med J. 1972;130:38–53.
8. Forsberg JG. Cervicovaginal epithelium: its origin and development. Am J Obstet Gynecol. 1973;115:1025–43.
9. Morcel K, Guerrier D, Watrin T, Pellerin I, Leveque J. The Mayer-Rokitansky-Küster-Hauser (MRKH) syndrome: clinical description and genetics. J Gynecol Obstet Biol Reprod. 2008;37(6):539–46.
10. Mortlock DP, Innis JW. Mutation of HOXA13 in hand-foot-genital syndrome. Nat Genet. 1997;15(2):179–80.
11. Lalwani S, Wu HH, Reindollar RH, Gray MR. HOXA10 mutations in congenital absence of uterus and vagina. Fertil Steril. 2008;89(2):325–30.
12. Oppelt P, Renner SP, Brucker S, Strissel PL, Strick R, Oppelt PG, et al. The VCUAM (Vagina Cervix Uterus Adnex-associated Malformation) classification: a new classification for genital malformations. Fertil Steril. 2005;84(5):1493–7.
13. Buttram VC Jr, Gibbons WE. Müllerian anomalies: a proposed classification. (An analysis of 144 cases). Fertil Steril. 1979;32(1):40–6.
14. Grimbizis GF, Gordts S, Di Spiezio Sardo A, Brucker S, De Angelis C, Gergolet M, et al. The ESHRE/ESGE consensus on the classification of female genital tract congenital anomalies. Hum Reprod. 2013;28:2032–44.
15. Morcel K, Camborieux L. Programme de Recherches sur les Aplasies Mülleriennes, Guerrier D. Mayer-Rokitansky-Kuster-Hauser (MRKH) syndrome. Orphanet J Rare Dis. 2007;2:13.
16. Herlin M, Bjorn AM, Rasmussen M, Trolle B, Petersen MB. Prevalence and patient characteristics of Mayer-Rokitansky-Kuster-Hauser syndrome: a Nationwide registry-based study. Hum Reprod. 2016;31:2384–90.
17. Timmreck LS, Reindollar RH. Contemporary issues in primary amenorrhea. Obstet Gynecol Clin N Am. 2003;30:287–302.
18. Zhang Y, Chen Y, Hua K. Outcomes in patients undergoing robotic reconstructive uterovaginal anastomosis of congenital cervical and vaginal atresia. Int J Med Robot Comput Assist Surg. 2017;13:1821.
19. Letterie GS. Management of congenital uterine abnormalities. Reprod Biomed Online. 2011;23(1):40–52.
20. Reichman D, Laufer MR, Robinson BK. Pregnancy outcomes in unicornuate uteri: a review. Fertil Steril. 2009;91:1886–94.
21. Kapczuk K, Friebe Z, Iwaniec K, Kedzia W. Obstructive müllerian anomalies in menstruating adolescent girls: a report of 22 cases. J Pediatr Adolesc Gynecol. 2018;31(3):252–7.

22. Yoo R-E, Cho JY, Kim SY, Kim SH. A systematic approach to the magnetic resonance imaging-based differential diagnosis of congenital Müllerian duct anomalies and their mimics. Abdom Imaging. 2014;40(1):192–206.
23. Valle RF, Ekpo GE. Hysteroscopic metroplasty for the septate uterus: review and meta-analysis. J Minim Invasive Gynecol. 2013;20(1):22–42.
24. Kaufman RH, Adan E, Binder GL, Gerthoffer F. Upper genital tract changes and pregnancy outcome in offspring exposed in utero to diethylstilbestrol. Am J Obstet Gynecol. 1980;137:299.
25. Williams CE, Nakhal RS, Hall-Craggs MA, Wood D, Cutner A, Pattison SH, et al. Transverse vaginal septae: management and long-term outcomes. BJOG. 2014;121:1653–9.
26. Grimbizis GF, Di Spiezio Sardo A, Saravelos SH, Gordts S, Exacoustos C, Van Schoubroeck D, et al. The Thessaloniki ESHRE/ESGE consensus on diagnosis of female genital anomalies. Hum Reprod. 2016;31(1):2–7.
27. Nicolini U, Bellotti M, Bonazzi B, Zamberletti D, Candiani GB. Can ultrasound be used to screen uterine malformations? Fertil Steril. 1987;47:89–93.
28. Woodward PJ, Sohaey R, Wagner BJ. Congenital uterine malformations. Curr Probl Diagn Radiol. 1995;24:178–97.
29. Raga F, Bonilla-Musoles F, Blanes J, Osborne NG. Congenital Müllerian anomalies: diagnostic accuracy of three-dimensional ultrasound. Fertil Steril. 1996;65:523.
30. Troiano RN, McCarthy SM. Mullerian duct anomalies: imaging and clinical issues. Radiology. 2004;233:19.
31. Pellerito JS, McCarthy SM, Doyle MB, Glickman MG, DeCherney AH. Diagnosis of uterine anomalies: relative accuracy of MR imaging, endovaginal sonography, and hysterosalpingography. Radiology. 1992;183:795.
32. Olpin JD, Moeni A, Willmore RJ, Heilbrun ME. MR imaging of müllerian fusion anomalies. Magn Reson Imaging Clin N Am. 2017;25(3):563–75.
33. Goldberg JM, Falcone T, Attaran M. Sonohysterographic evaluation of uterine abnormalities noted on hysterosalpingography. Hum Reprod. 1997;12:2151–3.
34. Vahdat M, Sariri E, Kashanian M, Najmi Z, Mobasseri A, Marashi M, et al. Can combination of hysterosalpingography and ultrasound replace hysteroscopy in diagnosis of uterine malformations in infertile women? Med J Islam Repub Iran. 2016;30:352.
35. Buttram VC. Mullerian anomalies and their management. Fertil Steril. 1983;40:159.
36. Salim R, Regan L, Woelfer B, Backos M, Jurkovic D. A comparative study of the morphology of congenital uterine anomalies in women with and without a history of recurrent first trimester miscarriage. Hum Reprod. 2003;18:162–6.
37. Ludwin A, Ludwin I, Kudla M, Kottner J. Reliability of the European Society of Human Reproduction and Embryology/European Society for Gynaecological Endoscopy and American Society for Reproductive Medicine classification systems for congenital uterine anomalies detected using three-dimensional ultrasonography. Fertil Steril. 2015;104:688–97.
38. Woelfer B, Salim R, Banerjee S, Elson J, Regan L, Jurkovic D. Reproductive outcomes in women with congenital uterine anomalies detected by three-dimensional ultrasound screening. Obstet Gynecol. 2001;98:1099–103.
39. Ludwin A, Ludwin I. Comparison of the ESHRE-ESGE and ASRM classifications of mullerian duct anomalies in everyday practice. Hum Reprod. 2015;30:569–80.
40. Ludwin A, Ludwin I, Pitynski K, Banas T, Jach R. Role of morphologic characteristics of the uterine septum in the prediction and prevention of abnormal healing outcomes after hysteroscopic metroplasty. Hum Reprod. 2014;29:1420–31.
41. Knez J, Saridogan E, van den Bosch T, Mavrelos D, Ambler G, Jurkovic D. ESHRE/ESGE female genital tract anomalies classification system—the potential impact of discarding arcuate uterus on clinical practice. Hum Reprod. 2018;33:600–6.
42. Prior M, Richardson A, Asif S, Polanski L, Parris-Larkin M, Chandler J, et al. Outcome of assisted reproduction in women with congenital uterine anomalies: a prospective observational study. Ultrasound Obstet Gynecol. 2018;51:110–7.
43. Bhagavath B, Ellie G, Griffiths KM, Winter T, Alur-Gupta S, Richardson C, et al. Uterine malformations: an update of diagnosis, management, and outcomes. Obstet Gynecol Surv. 2017;72:377–9.

44. Ludwin A, Martins WP, Nastri CO, Ludwin I, Coelho Neto MA, Leitao VM, et al. Congenital Uterine Malformation by Experts (CUME): better criteria for distinguishing between normal/arcuate and septate uterus? Ultrasound Obstet Gynecol. 2018;51:101–9.
45. Muasher SJ, Acosta AA, Garcia JE, Rosenwaks Z, Jones HW. Wedge metroplasty for the septate uterus: an update. Fertil Steril. 1984;42:515–9.
46. McShane PM, Reilly RJ, Schiff I. Pregnancy outcomes following Tompkins metroplasty. Fertil Steril. 1983;40:190–4.
47. Querleu D, Brasme TL, Parmentier D. Ultrasound-guided transcervical metroplasty. Fertil Steril. 1990;54:995–8.
48. Ghirardi V, Bizzarri N, Remorgida V, Venturini PL, Ferrero S. Intraoperative transrectal ultrasonography for hysteroscopic metroplasty: feasibility and safety. J Minim Invasive Gynecol. 2015;22:884–8.
49. Fedele L, Bianchi S. Hysteroscopic metroplasty for septate uterus. Obstet Gynecol Clin North Am. 1995;22:473.
50. Ludwin A, Ludwin I, Bhagavath B, Lindheim SR. Pre-, intra-, and postoperative management of Robert's uterus. Fertil Steril. 2018;110:778–9.
51. Jayasinghe Y, Rane A, Stalewski H, Grover S. The presentation and early diagnosis of the rudimentary uterine horn. Obstet Gynecol. 2005;105:1456.
52. Papp Z, Mezei G, Gavai M, Hupukizi P, Urbancsek J. Reproductive performance after transabdominal metroplasty: a review of 157 consecutive cases. J Reprod Med. 2006;51:544e52.
53. Davies MC, Creighton SM, Woodhouse CRJ. The pitfalls of vaginal construction. BJU Int. 2005;95:1293–8.
54. Creatsas G, Deligeoroglou E, Christopoulos P. Creation of a neovagina after Creatsas modification of Williams vaginoplasty for the treatment of 200 patients with Mayer-Rokitansky-Kuster-Hauser syndrome. Fertil Steril. 2010;94(5):1848–52.
55. Creatsas G, Deligeoroglou E. Expert opinion: vaginal aplasia: creation of a neovagina following the Creatsas vaginoplasty. Eur J Obstet Gynecol Reprod Biol. 2007;131(2):248–52.
56. Creatsas G, Deligeoroglou E. Vaginal aplasia and reconstruction. Best Pract Res Clin Obstet Gynaecol. 2010;24(2):185–91.
57. Laggari V, Diareme S, Christogiorgos S, Deligeoroglou E, Christopoulos P, Tsiantis J, Creatsas G. Anxiety and depression in adolescents with polycystic ovary syndrome and Mayer-Rokitansky-Kuster-Hauser syndrome. J Psychosom Obstet Gynaecol. 2009;30(2):83–8.
58. Adamyan LV. Laparoscopic management of vaginal aplasia with or without functional noncommunicating rudimentary uterus. In: Arregui ME, Fitzgibbons Jr RJ, Katkhouda N, McKernan JB, Reich H, editors. Principles of laparoscopic surgery: basic and advanced techniques. New York: Springer; 1995. p. 646–51.
59. Davydov SN, Zhvitiashvili OD. Formation of vagina (colpopoiesis) from peritoneum of Douglas pouch. Acta Chir Plast. 1974;16:35–41.
60. Adamyan LV. Therapeutic and endoscopic perspectives. In: Nichols DH, Clarke-Pearson DL, editors. Gynecologic, obstetric, and related surgery. 2nd ed. St. Louis: Mosby; 2000. p. 1209–17.
61. Allen LM, Lucco KL, Brown CM, Spitzer RF, Kives S. Psychosexual and functional outcomes after creation of a neovagina with laparoscopic Davydov in patients with vaginal agenesis. Fertil Steril. 2010;94:2272–6.
62. Brånnstrom M. Womb transplants with live births: an update and the future. €. Expert Opin Biol Ther. 2017;17:1105–12.
63. Wei L, Xue T, Tao KS, Zhang G, Zhao GY, Yu SQ, et al. Modified human uterus transplantation using ovarian veins for venous drainage: the first report of surgically successful robotic-assisted uterus procurement and follow-up for 12 months. Fertil Steril. 2017;108:346–56.
64. Dillon W, Mudaliar N, Wingate M. Congenital atresia of the cervix. Obstet Gynecol. 1979;54:126–9.
65. Fujimoto VY, Miller JH, Klein NA, Soules MR. Congenital cervical atresia: report of seven cases and review of the literature. Am J Obstet Gynecol. 1997;177:1419–25.

66. Rock JA, Roberts CP, Jones HW. Congenital anomalies of the uterine cervix: lessons from 30 cases managed clinically a common protocol. Fertil Steril. 2010;94:1858–63.
67. Casey CA, Laufer MR. Cervical agenesis: septic death after surgery. Obstet Gynecol. 1997;90:706–7.
68. Deffarges JV, Haddad I, Musset R, Paniel BJ. Utero-vaginal anastomosis in women with uterine cervix atresia: long-term follow-up and reproductive performance. A study of 18 cases. Hum Reprod. 2001;16:1772–5.
69. Kriplani A, Kachhawa G, Awasthi D, Kulsherestha V. Laparoscopic-assisted uterovaginal anastomosis in congenital atresia of uterine cervix: follow-up study. J Minim Invasive Gynecol. 2012;19:477–84.
70. Rikken JFW, Kowalik CR, Emanuel MH, Bongers MY, Spinder T, de Kruif JH, et al. The randomised uterine septum transsection trial (TRUST): design and protocol. BMC Womens Health. 2018;18:163.
71. Parsanezhad ME, Alborzi S, Zarei A, Dehbashi S, Shirzai LG, Rajaeefard A, et al. Hysteroscopic metroplasty of the complete uterine septum, duplicate cervix, and vaginal septum. Fertil Steril. 2006;85:1473–7.
72. Grynberg M, Gervaise A, Faivre E, Deffieux X, Frydman R, Fernandez H. Treatment of twenty-two patients with complete uterine and vaginal septum. J Minim Invasive Gynecol. 2012;19:34–9.
73. Fedele L, Motta F, Frontino G, Restelli E, Bianchi S. Double uterus with obstructed hemivagina and ipsilateral renal agenesis: pelvic anatomic variants in 87 cases. Hum Reprod. 2013;28:1580–3.
74. Smith NA, Laufer MR. Obstructed hemivagina and ipsilateral renal anomaly (OHVIRA) syndrome: management and follow-up. Fertil Steril. 2007;87:918–22.
75. Tong J, Zhu L, Lang J. Clinical characteristics of 70 patients with Herlyn-Werner-Wunderlich syndrome. Int J Gynecol Obstet. 2013;121:173–5.
76. Christiansen OB, Nybo Andersen AM, Bosch E, Daya S, Delves PJ, Hviid TV, et al. Evidence-based investigations and treatments of recurrent pregnancy loss. Fertil Steril. 2005;83:821–39.
77. Kowalik CR, Goddijn M, Emanuel MH, Bongers MY, Spinder T, de Kruif JH, et al. Metroplasty versus expectant management for women with recurrent miscarriage and a septate uterus. Cochrane Database Syst Rev. 2011:CD008576.
78. Rikken JF, Kowalik CR, Emanuel MH, Mol BW, van der Veen F, van Wely M, et al. Septum resection for women of reproductive age with a septate uterus. Cochrane Database Syst Rev. 2017:CD008576.

Adolescent Amenorrhea: New Aspects of an Old Problem

Laura Gaspari, Françoise Paris, Nicolas Kalfa, Samir Hamamah, and Charles Sultan

Primary amenorrhea (PA), which occurs in 1–5% of girls, describes complete absence of menses, and it is a devastating diagnosis that can affect an adolescent view of her feminity, sexuality, fertility, and self-image [1].

A prompt confirmation of the diagnosis is mandatory. When necessary, estrogen replacement treatment should be advised for pubertal development and psychological improvement [2].

Assessment of adolescent patients requires a sensitive, age-appropriated approach, considering the emotional maturity of the adolescent distress.

L. Gaspari · F. Paris
Unité d'Endocrinologie-Gynécologie Pédiatrique, Service de Pédiatrie, CHU Montpellier, University of Montpellier, Montpellier, France

Centre de Référence Maladies Rares du Développement Génital, Constitutif Sud, CHU Montpellier, University of Montpellier, Montpellier, France

INSERM 1203, Développement Embryonnaire Fertilité Environnement, University of Montpellier, Montpellier, France

N. Kalfa
Centre de Référence Maladies Rares du Développement Génital, Constitutif Sud, CHU Montpellier, University of Montpellier, Montpellier, France

Département de Chirurgie Viscérale et Urologique Pédiatrique, CHU Montpellier, University of Montpellier, Montpellier, France

S. Hamamah
INSERM 1203, Développement Embryonnaire Fertilité Environnement, University of Montpellier, Montpellier, France

Département de Biologie de la Reproduction, Biologie de la Reproduction/DPI et CECOS, CHU Montpellier, University of Montpellier, Montpellier, France

C. Sultan (✉)
Unité d'Endocrinologie-Gynécologie Pédiatrique, Service de Pédiatrie, CHU Montpellier, University of Montpellier, Montpellier, France

© International Society of Gynecological Endocrinology 2023
A. R. Genazzani et al. (eds.), *Amenorrhea*, ISGE Series,
https://doi.org/10.1007/978-3-031-22378-5_2

Moreover, cultural perceptions and practices around menarche and adolescent menstruation vary among countries, groups, and ethnics. Menstruation can be described as a Dr. Jekyll and Hyde phenomenon! It carries both a good and a bad reputation: a "good reputation" since menarche is important as a sign of maturity and fertility, and a "bad reputation" due to the persistence of physical and psychological problems.

PA in adolescence is likely to require a multidisciplinary input including that of a pediatric endocrinologist, a gynecologist, a surgeon, a clinical psychologist, and a fertility team.

It is generally accepted that the menstrual cycle is a biological marker of general health in adolescents. Although pubertal menstrual disorders, such as oligomenorrhea, dysfunctional uterine bleeding, and amenorrhea, commonly occur within the 2 years after menarche, prolonged amenorrhea beyond 14 years is not normal and needs management.

Facing an adolescent with PA should raise four questions:

- Why should amenorrhea be considered as a "vital" sign?
- Who should be evaluated for amenorrhea?
- How should adolescent amenorrhea be evaluated?
- What are the causes of adolescent amenorrhea?

2.1   Why Should Amenorrhea Be Considered as a "Vital" Sign?

PA provides a window of opportunity for early diagnosis/treatment of conditions affecting hypothalamic-pituitary-ovarian (HPO) axis [3]. It may be associated with significant medical morbidity and may offer the opportunity of early identification of potential health concerns for adulthood [4].

PA is a risk factor for early and late consequences, according to the degree of estrogenization.

In estrogen-repleted adolescents, peri-pubertal hyperestrogenism constitutes a risk for hyperplasia of the endometrium, responsible for dysfunctional uterine bleeding and, later, a risk for endometrial cancer and breast cancer. Conversely, in estrogen-deficient adolescents, reduction of bone mineral density increases the lifelong risk of fractures [5] and cardiovascular risk is increased in this condition. In addition, psychological problems, and even psychiatric disorders, should not be overlooked.

2.2   Who Should Be Evaluated for Amenorrhea?

There is no consensus regarding the type of PA that requires investigations. In our experience, management of PA should start in four conditions:

- An adolescent who has not had menarche by age 14 years
- An adolescent who has not had menarche and more than 3 years have elapsed since thelarche
- An adolescent who has not had a menarche by age 13 years and no secondary sexual development
- An adolescent who has not had menarche by age 14 years and there is a suspicion of an eating disorder or excessive exercise, or there are signs of hyperandrogenism, or there is evidence of a failure to thrive.

2.3   How Should Adolescent Amenorrhea Be Evaluated?

In the presence of an adolescent girl with PA, diagnosis can be oriented with the aid of history, physical examination, imaging studies, hormonal evaluation, and karyotyping [1]:

(a) Evaluation of PA begins with a thorough medical history, general health, and lifestyles, to identify chronic illness and exposure to radiations or chemotherapy during infancy. Any history of galactorrhea, headache, and cyclic abdominal pain may be indicative [6].

(b) Physical examination includes height and weight and BMI. Breast Tanner staging is a good marker of the degree of estrogenization [7]. Any features of Turner syndrome must be looked for. A scrupulous examination of the external genitalia should be conducted, along with a normal cervix [2].

(c) Imaging studies routinely include pelvic ultrasonography to confirm the presence of ovaries and the uterus.

(d) Initial hormonal evaluation is limited to the serum FSH (and LH), testosterone, and prolactin levels [8]. Pregnancy must be rolled out, since adolescents may ovulate before the first period. A karyotype should be conducted in all adolescents with high FSH serum levels.

At the end of this evaluation, the causes of PA should be discussed (Fig. 2.1):

- According to the initial examination: PA with or without breast development, with or without evidence of androgen excess, with or without galactorrhea, with or without weight loss, with or without growth failure
- According to the FSH levels: hypergonadotropic hypogonadism (elevated FSH), hypogonadotropic hypogonadism (low FSH), or eugonadism (normal FSH)
- According to karyotype: XX, XO, or XY [9]

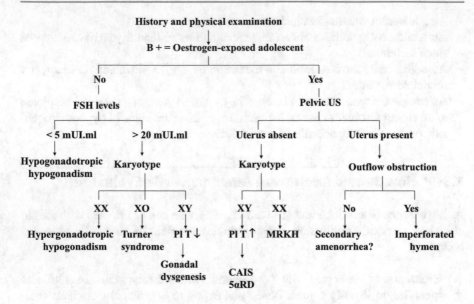

Fig. 2.1 Algorithm for the evaluation of primary amenorrhea. Abbreviation: *Pl T* plasma testosterone level, *MRKH* Mayer-Rokitansky-Küster-Hauser syndrome, *CAIS* complete androgen insensitivity syndrome, *5αR* 5α-reductase

2.4   What Are the Causes of Adolescent Amenorrhea?

According to the practice committee of the American Society for Reproductive Medicine, PA may be associated with anatomic defects of the outflow tract, primary hypogonadism (XX, X0, XY), hypothalamic causes (dysfunctional, Kallmann, chronic illness), pituitary causes (prolactinoma, illness), other endocrine gland disorders (adrenal, thyroid, ovary), and multifactorial causes (PCOS). This classification in our opinion does not reflect the routine practice. We prefer to consider that PA could be related to endocrine defects within the hypothalamic-pituitary-ovarian axis, genetic abnormalities, previous radio- or chemotherapy, metabolic disease, autoimmune disorders, infections, contamination by endocrine-disrupting chemicals (EDCs), Mullerian defects, or unknown factors.

In our experience, during the last decades, causes of PA have been anatomic defects of the outflow tract (10%), ovarian causes (30%), pituitary causes (5%), hypothalamic causes (10%), functional causes (30%), and idiopathic causes (30–35%).

The main causes of PA are considered to be related to:

1. Endocrine defects within the hypothalamic-pituitary-ovarian axis
2. Genetic defects of the ovary
3. Metabolic diseases
4. Autoimmune diseases
5. Infections

6. Iatrogenic causes (radiotherapy, chemotherapy)
7. Mullerian defects
8. Environmental factors
9. Idiopathic factors

2.4.1 Endocrine Defects Within the Hypothalamic-Pituitary-Ovarian Axis (Table 2.1)

When puberty does not occur at the extreme end of the normal spectrum (i.e., constitutional delay of growth and puberty), hypogonadism must be evaluated. There are two types of hypogonadism: hypogonadotropic hypogonadism and hypergonadotropic hypogonadism. Hypogonadotropic hypogonadism can be transient due to an underlying medical condition, or persistent due to a GnRH defect. Midline congenital defects, such as cleft lip and palate, and neural tube defects are suggestive of permanent hypogonadotropic hypogonadism. Hypergonadotropic hypogonadism is due to gonadal failure.

2.4.1.1 Hypogonadotropic Hypogonadism

Hypogonadotropic hypogonadism may be congenital and due to isolated FSH-LH deficiency or multiple gonadotropic deficiency. It may be secondary to acquired hypothalamic-pituitary disease. Hypothalamic-pituitary diseases include Kallmann syndrome, Prader-Willi syndrome, congenital hypopituitarism, and septo-optic dysplasia, among others.

Table 2.1 Endocrine defects within the hypothalamic-pituitary-ovarian axis

Hypogonadotropic hypogonadism		
Congenital	GnRH deficiencies and anosmia (Kallmann syndrome)	
	Syndromic (Prader-Willi syndrome, CHARGE syndrome, Laurence-Moon syndrome, …)	
Acquired	Pituitary adenoma	
	Infiltrative disorders (histiocytosis, sarcoidosis, hemochromatosis, …)	
	Brain trauma	
	Radiation	
	Drugs	
Hypergonadotropic hypogonadism		
XO	Turner syndrome	
XX	Congenital premature ovarian insufficiency (genetic defect)	
	Acquired	Infections
		Radiotherapy, chemotherapy
		Autoimmune diseases
XY	Gonadal dysgenesis	
	Testosterone biosynthesis defects	
	Androgen resistance (CAIS, 5αRD)	

Abbreviation: *CAIS* complete androgen insensitivity syndrome, *5αRD* 5α-reductase deficiency

Congenital Hypogonadotropic Hypogonadism

Hypogonadotropic hypogonadism may be due to genetic abnormalities. Recognizing these gene variations may improve our diagnosis capabilities:

- GnRH receptors, KISS1/KISS1R and TAC3/TACR3, should be the first genes to be screened in a clinical setting for equivocal cases such as DP versus IHH, since they are the main causes of GnRH pulse generator defects.
- In Kallmann syndrome, genetic screening for particular genes should be prioritized based on the association of specific clinical features: synkinesis (KAL1), dental agenesis (FGF8/FGFR1), bone anomalies (FGF8/FGFR1), and hearing loss (CHD7, SOX1). New genes have recently been identified, and the list of genes involved in hypogonadotropic hypogonadism is still growing.

More than 25 different genes have been implicated in congenital hypogonadotropic hypogonadism and/or Kallmann syndrome, which account for about 50% of cases.

Acquired Hypogonadotropic Hypogonadism

Absence of maturation of the hypothalamic-pituitary-ovarian axis may be secondary to acquired hypothalamic-pituitary disease, such as:

- Brain tumor: craniopharyngioma, astrocytoma
- Infiltration diseases of the CNS: histiocytosis
- Chemo- or radiotherapy
- Hyperprolactinemia

2.4.1.2   Hypergonadotropic Hypogonadism

Hypergonadotropic hypogonadism may be congenital or acquired.
    According to the karyotype, one can distinguish:

- XX hypergonadotropic hypogonadism: premature ovarian insufficiency. Premature ovarian insufficiency (POI) affects about 1/10,000 adolescent girls and is characterized by severe estrogen deficiency due to ovarian dysgenesis, which can be congenital or acquired. This aspect will be treated in the next section.
- X0 hypergonadotropic hypogonadism: Turner syndrome. Turner syndrome (TS) is the most prevalent example of hypergonadotropic hypogonadism. Although 20% of TS patients will begin puberty spontaneously, only a small minority will progress to menarche. Absent puberty and PA are very frequent clinical expressions of TS. In most TS cases, primary ovarian failure can be expected.
- XY hypergonadotropic hypogonadism: disorders of sex development (DSD). 46,XY DSD refers to 46,XY adolescents with undermasculinization, leading in some cases to a female phenotype. The first estimate on the prevalence of 46,XY females is 6.4 per 100,000 live-born females in Denmark [10]. The hormonal levels of T, AMH, FSH, and LH, as well as the presence of Mullerian derivatives

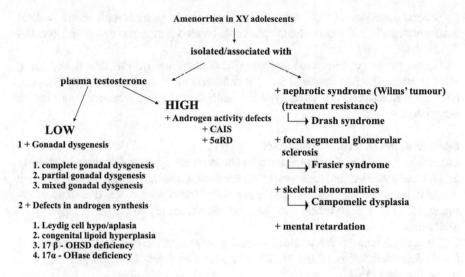

Fig. 2.2 Main causes of XY adolescent amenorrhea. Abbreviation: *17β-OHSD* 17β-hydroxysteroid dehydrogenase, *17α-OHase* 17α-hydroxylase, *CAIS* complete androgen insensitivity syndrome, *5αRD* 5α-reductase deficiency

noted by pelvic ultrasound, will differentiate gonadal dysgenesis (associated with insufficient gonadal secretion of T and AMH) from androgen production defects or androgen resistance (Fig. 2.2).

Gonadal Dysgenesis

Gonadal dysgenesis is a genetic defect in testis determination characterized by a variable alteration in Leydig and Sertoli cell function. This disorder may be secondary to mutations in any of the several genes taking part in the differentiation process of the primitive gonad to a testis.

SRY gene abnormalities express with a clinical picture of 46,XY sex reversal with female phenotype. The diagnosis of Swyer syndrome is made in the pubertal period in the presence of PA [11].

About 80% of the cases of gonadal dysgenesis are not caused by a SRY gene abnormality. They may be secondary to abnormalities in the other genes that take part in testis determination, however, and they are autosomal or X-linked.

Some cases of gonadal dysgenesis have been linked to SF1 gene mutation. This gene is involved in the development of male gonads and adrenal glands.

In some patients, gonadal dysgenesis is associated with renal dysfunction. In these cases, the diagnosis of Drash syndrome—defined as Wilms' tumor associated with renal insufficiency or Frasier syndrome, which is proteinuria secondary to focal glomerular sclerosis—may be made. Both syndromes are due to WT1 gene abnormalities that are nevertheless quite specific for each syndrome. In particular, heterozygous mutations in the open reading frame have been associated with Drash syndrome, while intron mutations leading to splicing abnormalities have been found in Frasier patients.

Several mutations of SOX-9 have been identified in patients with severe skeletal malformations like campomelic dysplasia, associated with sex reversal and gonadal dysgenesis.

Homozygous or composite heterozygous mutations of the desert hedgehog (DHH) gene, which is involved in testis differentiation and perineal development, have been identified. The phenotype is usually female, and a neuropathy may be associated.

Defects in Testosterone Production

Defects in T production are rare and are characterized by severe degrees of external genital undervirilization. Conversely, no Mullerian derivatives are present because AMH is normally secreted by the Sertoli cells. These defects are due to an enzymatic defect in T biosynthesis, or they may be secondary to an LH receptor gene abnormality.

Defect in 3-beta-hydroxysteroid dehydrogenase is associated with a variable but insufficient virilization of the 46,XY male, ranging from a female phenotype to minor forms of DSD.

The phenotype in cases of a 17-alpha-hydroxylase defect may also be extremely variable. In some individuals, the diagnosis is made only in the pubertal period because of PA. An excess of 11-deoxycorticosterone (DOC) causes hypertension during puberty. The genetic abnormality concerns the CYP17 gene with recessive transmission.

Defect of 17-beta-hydroxysteroid reductase is a rare testicular block that causes a deficit in testicular T production. The phenotype is more frequently female.

Leydig cell agenesis or hypoplasia is a rare form of 46,XY DSD, first identified in a patient with female phenotype associated with the 46,XY karyotype. The patient presented primary amenorrhea and no breast development at puberty, associated with low T at baseline and after hCG stimulation testing. This condition is determined by a homozygous or double-heterozygous inactivating mutation of the LH receptor gene.

Androgen Resistance Disorders

The androgen resistance disorders are characterized by normal/high T and AMH production, in contrast to the undermasculinization in 46,XY DSD. These disorders are represented by androgen receptor defect or 5α-reductase deficiency.

Complete Androgen Insensitivity Syndrome (CAIS)

The diagnosis of CAIS is often made in the pubertal period, when primary amenorrhea associated with normal breast development and sparse axillary and pubic hair suggests this diagnosis [12]. The endocrine investigations show high plasma T, along with a high LH level. An AR gene mutation will confirm this diagnosis.

5aR Deficiency

In the case of 5aR deficiency, T is not converted to dihydrotestosterone (DHT), which is responsible for external genital virilization. The phenotype is usually female, but it may assume all degrees of undervirilization [13, 14]. It is usually made at puberty because of PA, absence of breast development, striking virilization including hirsutism, clitoral hypertrophy, significant muscle development, and a masculinization in behavior. The molecular investigation confirms the diagnosis by identifying a 5aR2 gene mutation.

In conclusion, the XY adolescent referred for DP encompasses a wide variety of endocrine and genetic disorders. This complex situation requires a multidisciplinary team for diagnostic investigations, gender choice, treatment, and psychological management.

2.4.2 Genetic Defects of Ovary

Genetic O causes of PA include X chromosome alterations and autosomal gene abnormalities.

2.4.2.1 X Chromosome
X chromosome alterations include X chromosome monosomy X0, mosaicism XX and X0, X deletions, and translocations. In a recent work, Ghosh et al. reported that chromosomal anomalies contribute to be one of the major etiologies of amenorrhea, in India [15]. Besides, BMP-15 mutations and pre-mutation of the FMR1 gene (fragile X syndrome) are present in about 20% of adolescents with PA.

Turner syndrome (TS) is associated with X chromosome numerical or structural alterations. Prevalence of TS is about 50/100,000 females in Caucasian population. Ovarian dysgenesis and early follicular apoptosis are key features of TS, resulting in primary ovarian insufficiency with estrogen deficiency in the peri-pubertal period [16]. AMH plasma level can be useful as a marker of ovarian function.

2.4.2.2 Autosomal Gene Mutations
The prevalence of known genetic alterations that may be linked to PA is estimated to be around 20%. To date, 18 known primary ovarian insufficiency genes have been identified: BMP15, DMC1, EIF2S2, FIGLA, FOXL2, FSHR, GDF9, GPR3, HFM1, LHX8, MSH5, NOBOX, NR5A1, PGRMC1, STAG3, XPNPEP2, BHLB, and FSHB.

In a recent work, Eskenazi et al. reported, by the next-generation sequencing of these genes, that 25% of adolescents with PA presented at least one variant, and 18% presented a variant of unknown signification. In this study, NOBOX was the most common gene variant (19% of the patients) [17].

2.4.3 Metabolic Disorders

- Classic galactosemia affects 5–25,000 female newborns and is due to mutation of the GALT gene, decreasing/abolishing galactose-1-phosphate uridylyltrans-ferase (GALT) activity, leading to toxic accumulation of galactose in the ovary as well as in the whole body. Direct toxicity of galactose is due to an accelerated atresia of the ovarian follicular pool. Several mechanisms have been postulated, including direct toxicity of galactose to oocytes and follicles, leading to accelerated atresia of the ovarian pool [18]. In animal studies, impaired primordial germ cell development has been reported.

- Thalassemia and sickle cell disease are the most prevalent inherited recessive hemoglobin disorders. Transfusion-related iron overload may lead to gonadal dysfunction and absence of pubertal development along with PA [19].
- Other metabolic disorders may also be associated with PA, such as congenial adrenal hyperplasia, due to 17-hydroxylase enzyme deficiency and aromatase deficiency. In some cases, type 1 diabetes through low BMI and abnormal pulsatile GnRH secretion may be related to PA.
- Obesity: Severe obese adolescents usually have elevated levels of plasma androgens. Normalization of plasma androgens by weight loss, which leads to resumption of ovulation, suggests that overweight-related hyperandrogenism is a cause of amenorrhea in obese adolescent girls. It is not rare that PA may reveal polycystic ovarian syndrome, especially when severe insulin resistance is present in the peri-pubertal period [20, 21].
- Lactational amenorrhea: Accessibility and availability of contraceptive for adolescents in low-income and middle-income countries are problematic [22]. Besides interruption of contraceptive supplies and lack of financial affordability, religious and social pressures prevent millions of adolescents from obtaining contraception in Africa, Latin America, and Asia. Although it does not directly concern adolescents with amenorrhea per se, the period of postpartum amenorrhea can be prolonged by breast-feeding [23].

2.4.4 Autoimmune Diseases

Autoimmune disease is the second most common disorder, associated with diabetes mellitus, hypothyroidism, Hashimoto thyroiditis, and Graves' disease. Autoimmune poly-endocrinopathy syndrome may also be associated with PA [24].

Evidence for autoimmune mechanisms involved in primary ovarian insufficiency is based on lymphocytic oophoritis, associated with autoantibodies to ovarian antigens [25]. Association with other autoimmune disorders of adrenal gland, thyroid, and pancreas is well known. A well-defined form of autoimmune diseases associated with PA is the autoimmune polyglandular form (APS) caused by a mutation of the AIRE gene. Besides, autoimmune disorders can be associated with non-endocrine diseases, such as candidiasis, vitiligo, systemic lupus, and rheumatoid arthritis.

2.4.5 Infections

Young women living with HIV are 70% more likely to experience amenorrhea.

The overall prevalence of amenorrhea among women with HIV infection is around 5%. In a recent meta-analysis, King et al. showed a significant association between HIV and amenorrhea with OR of 1.68 [26]. It is unclear whether amenorrhea might be a complication of HIV infection itself or due to other risk factors, such as low BMI, wasting (collapse of GhRH secretion), opiate and antipsychotic use (anovulation), immunosuppression, and chemotherapy. According to Cejtin et al., amenorrhea is reversible in 37% of cases [27].

2.4.6   Iatrogenic Causes (Radiotherapy, Chemotherapy)

Modern pediatric cancer treatment regimens are becoming highly effective, so the monitoring of endocrine and gynecological consequences in the adolescent cancer survivors is imperative [28, 29]. The prevalence of ovarian failure was considered around 10%, while Jablonska et al. reported that 31.6% of cancer survivors experience amenorrhea [30]. Actually, there is a wide range of ovarian insufficiency in survivors of pediatric cancers, ranging from 2.1 to 92.2% [31].

Within the ovarian follicles, both oocytes and granulosa cells are vulnerable to damage caused by chemotherapy. In addition, damage to blood vessels and focal fibrosis of the ovarian cortex are involved in chemotherapy-induced ovarian damage [32].

Besides chemotherapy with alkylating agents, abdominal pelvic radiation must be considered as a risk factor. It is well demonstrated that the AMH plasma level is a good marker of ovarian reserve [33]. Adolescents treated with total body irradiation (TBI) before stem cell transplant presented undetectable AMH [34]. Oocytes are very sensitive to radiotherapy. The detrimental effects depend on irradiation field, dosage, and fractionation schedules. Children cancer survivors, who received radiotherapy to the abdomen, pelvis, and total body, have lower AMH level [35].

Besides, following pediatric brain injury, endocrine dysfunction may include PA [36].

2.4.7   Mullerian Defects

Mullerian anomalies affect up to 4–5% of females [37]. Several classifications have been proposed without consensus. The most used and accepted one is proposed by the ASRM, which separates the anomalies in 12 classes [38].

Congenital malformation of the female genital organs includes absence of uterus and vagina and some obstructive abnormalities of the reproductive tract [39]. Mullerian aplasia or hypoplasia also known as Mayer-Rokitansky-Küster-Hauser syndrome may be isolated or associated with other congenital malformations [40].

Transverse vaginal septum is caused by persistence of the vaginal plate after it meets the Mullerian tract. Examination reveals a shortened blind vaginal pouch.

Imperforated hymen usually presents as a bluish bulging mass due to hematocolpos at the entrance of the vagina.

2.4.8   Environmental Factors (Lifestyle, Endocrine Disruptors)

Many EDCs are known to target the ovary, focusing their effects on both folliculo-genesis and steroidogenesis during the fetal life [41]. Several experimental data demonstrated the harmful effects of EDCs in the development of follicular growth through an acceleration of atresia [42]. Besides, some EDCs, such as pesticides, phthalates, bisphenol A, and dioxin, are known to compromise ovarian steroidogen-esis. Severe acute and chronic prenatal exposure to EDC may thus impair ovarian function later in life and disturb pubertal development [43].

2.4.9   Idiopathic

In the past, concealment of diagnosis and treatment information from patients was the standard practice. It is now an established practice to disclose the diagnosis and its etiology. This is usually gradually done in adolescence, depending on the level of understanding and knowledge. Disclosure of diagnosis allows better compliance with medical treatment and allows for other members of the family to be screened.

2.5   Treatment

The overall goal of estrogen replacement therapy in girls with hypogonadism is to start the development and maturation of secondary sexual characteristics and uter-ine growth and ensure normal growth velocity and optimal bone mass acquisition as well as to reduce the psychological consequences [44].

The treatment of PA depends on the underlying causes, as well as the health status, psychological concerns, and goals of the patients.

Some authors propose a short-term test with a low dose of estrogen for 6–12 months (2–6 mg/day). Although there is no consensus about this procedure, we have followed this advice.

Pubertal estrogen replacement therapy has mainly been based on each personal experience since there was no consensus regarding the estrogen drug, treatment route, dose, and dosing time or tempo [45].

There are various treatment protocols: estrogen therapy is routinely initiated around the age of 12–13 years, at a low dose (approximately 1/10 of the adult dose), and gradually increased over 2–4 years. Transdermal estrogens (patch or gel) seem more physiological.

Regardless of the estrogen form, route, and dose, it is also crucial to introduce appropriate estrogen therapy to prepare patients for an assisted reproductive procedure.

In adult life, the most frequent therapeutic approach of infertility is embryo transfer from donated oocytes. Moreover, the reconstitution of complete oogenesis from induced pluripotent stem cells would prove helpful [46].

2.6   Conclusions

Primary amenorrhea can be due to endocrine, genetic, metabolic, anatomical, and environmental disorders that may have severe implications for reproductive disturbances later in life.

In some complex cases, a multidisciplinary team best manages adolescents: pediatric endocrinologists, gynecologists, genetics, surgeons, radiologists, psychologists ....

Delay in the evaluation (and treatment) of adolescent amenorrhea in some cases may contribute to reduced bone density and other long-term adverse health consequences.

XY female adolescents are non-exceptional conditions and should be managed in reference centers [47].

Next-generation sequencing should be proposed to every adolescents with amenorrhea and idiopathic primary ovarian insufficiency.

Environmental endocrine disruptor (EDC) contamination during fetal life, childhood, and adolescence is a potential risk factor for adolescent amenorrhea.

References

1. Klein DA, Paradise SL, Reeder RM. Amenorrhea: a systematic approach to diagnosis and management. Am Fam Physician. 2019;100(1):39–48.
2. Master-Hunter T, Heiman DL. Amenorrhea: evaluation and treatment. Am Fam Physician. 2006;73(8):1374–82.
3. Popat VB, Prodanov T, Calis KA, Nelson LM. The menstrual cycle: a biological marker of general health in adolescents. Ann N Y Acad Sci. 2008;1135:43–51.
4. American Academy of Pediatrics Committee on Adolescence, American College of Obstetricians, Gynecologists Committee on Adolescent Health Care, Diaz A, Laufer MR, Breech LL. Menstruation in girls and adolescents: using the menstrual cycle as a vital sign. Pediatrics. 2006;118(5):2245–50.
5. Gordon CM, Nelson LM. Amenorrhea and bone health in adolescents and young women. Curr Opin Obstet Gynecol. 2003;15(5):377–84.
6. Golden NH, Carlson JL. The pathophysiology of amenorrhea in the adolescent. Ann N Y Acad Sci. 2008;1135:163–78.
7. Yoon JY, Cheon CK. Evaluation and management of amenorrhea related to congenital sex hormonal disorders. Ann Pediatr Endocrinol Metab. 2019;24(3):149–57.
8. Practice Committee of American Society for Reproductive Medicine. Current evaluation of amenorrhea. Fertil Steril. 2008;90(5 Suppl):S219–25.
9. Lee Y, Kim C, Park Y, Pyun JA, Kwack K. Next generation sequencing identifies abnormal Y chromosome and candidate causal variants in premature ovarian failure patients. Genomics. 2016;108(5–6):209–15.
10. Berglund A, Johannsen TH, Stochholm K, Viuff MH, Fedder J, Main KM, et al. Incidence, prevalence, diagnostic delay, and clinical presentation of female 46,XY disorders of sex development. J Clin Endocrinol Metab. 2016;101(12):4532–40.
11. Meyer KF, Freitas Filho LG, Silva KI, Trauzcinsky PA, Reuter C, Souza MBM. The XY female and SWYER syndrome. Urol Case Rep. 2019;26:100939.
12. Sultan C, Lumbroso S, Paris F, Jeandel C, Terouanne B, Belon C, et al. Disorders of androgen action. Semin Reprod Med. 2002;20(3):217–28.

13. Maimoun L, Philibert P, Cammas B, Audran F, Bouchard P, Fenichel P, et al. Phenotypical, biological, and molecular heterogeneity of 5alpha-reductase deficiency: an extensive international experience of 55 patients. J Clin Endocrinol Metab. 2011;96(2):296–307.

14. Maimoun L, Philibert P, Bouchard P, Ocal G, Leheup B, Fenichel P, et al. Primary amenorrhea in four adolescents revealed 5alpha-reductase deficiency confirmed by molecular analysis. Fertil Steril. 2011;95(2):804.e1–5.

15. Ghosh S, Roy S, Halder A. Study of frequency and types of chromosomal abnormalities in phenotypically female patients with amenorrhea in Eastern Indian population. J Obstet Gynaecol Res. 2020;46(9):1627–38.

16. Trolle C, Mortensen KH, Hjerrild BE, Cleemann L, Gravholt CH. Clinical care of adult Turner syndrome—new aspects. Pediatr Endocrinol Rev. 2012;9(Suppl 2):739–49.

17. Eskenazi S, Bachelot A, Hugon-Rodin J, Plu-Bureau G, Gompel A, Catteau-Jonard S, et al. Next generation sequencing should be proposed to every woman with "idiopathic" primary ovarian insufficiency. J Endocr Soc. 2021;5(7):bvab032.

18. van Erven B, Berry GT, Cassiman D, Connolly G, Forga M, Gautschi M, et al. Fertility in adult women with classic galactosemia and primary ovarian insufficiency. Fertil Steril. 2017;108(1):168–74.

19. Mamsen LS, Kristensen SG, Pors SE, Botkjaer JA, Ernst E, Macklon KT, et al. Consequences of beta-thalassemia or sickle cell disease for ovarian follicle number and morphology in girls who had ovarian tissue cryopreserved. Front Endocrinol (Lausanne). 2020;11:593718.

20. Rachmiel M, Kives S, Atenafu E, Hamilton J. Primary amenorrhea as a manifestation of polycystic ovarian syndrome in adolescents: a unique subgroup? Arch Pediatr Adolesc Med. 2008;162(6):521–5.

21. Ledger WL, Skull J. Amenorrhoea: investigation and treatment. Curr Obstet Gynaecol. 2004;14:254–60.

22. Figaroa MNS, Bellizzi S, Delvaux T, Benova L. Lactational amenorrhoea among adolescent girls in low-income and middle-income countries: a systematic scoping review. BMJ Glob Health. 2020;5(10):e002492.

23. Abraha TH, Teferra AS, Gelagay AA, Welesamuel TG, Fisseha GK, Aregawi BG, et al. Knowledge and associated factors of lactational amenorrhea as a contraception method among postpartum women in Aksum town, Tigray Region, Ethiopia. BMC Res Notes. 2018;11(1):641.

24. Szeliga A, Calik-Ksepka A, Maciejewska-Jeske M, Grymowicz M, Smolarczyk K, Kostrzak A, et al. Autoimmune diseases in patients with premature ovarian insufficiency-our current state of knowledge. Int J Mol Sci. 2021;22(5):2594.

25. Komorowska B. Autoimmune premature ovarian failure. Prz Menopauzalny. 2016;15(4):210–4.

26. King EM, Albert AY, Murray MCM. HIV and amenorrhea: a meta-analysis. AIDS. 2019;33(3):483–91.

27. Cejtin HE, Evans CT, Greenblatt R, Minkoff H, Weber KM, Wright R, et al. Prolonged amenorrhea and resumption of menses in women with HIV. J Womens Health (Larchmt). 2018;27:1441.

28. van der Kooi ALF, Mulder RL, Hudson MM, Kremer LCM, Skinner R, Constine LS, et al. Counseling and surveillance of obstetrical risks for female childhood, adolescent, and young adult cancer survivors: recommendations from the International Late Effects of Childhood Cancer Guideline Harmonization Group. Am J Obstet Gynecol. 2021;224(1):3–15.

29. Beneventi F, Locatelli E, Giorgiani G, Zecca M, Locatelli F, Cavagnoli C, et al. Gonadal and uterine function in female survivors treated by chemotherapy, radiotherapy, and/ or bone marrow transplantation for childhood malignant and non-malignant diseases. BJOG. 2014;121(7):856–65; discussion 65.

30. Jablonska O, Shi Z, Valdez KE, Ting AY, Petroff BK. Temporal and anatomical sensitivities to the aryl hydrocarbon receptor agonist 2,3,7,8-tetrachlorodibenzo-p-dioxin leading to premature acyclicity with age in rats. Int J Androl. 2010;33(2):405–12.

31. Chemaitilly W, Li Z, Krasin MJ, Brooke RJ, Wilson CL, Green DM, et al. Premature ovarian insufficiency in childhood cancer survivors: a report from the St. Jude lifetime cohort. J Clin Endocrinol Metab. 2017;102(7):2242–50.

32. Gargus E, Deans R, Anazodo A, Woodruff TK. Management of primary ovarian insufficiency symptoms in survivors of childhood and adolescent cancer. J Natl Compr Cancer Netw. 2018;16(9):1137–49.
33. Lie Fong S, Laven JS, Hakvoort-Cammel FG, Schipper I, Visser JA, Themmen AP, et al. Assessment of ovarian reserve in adult childhood cancer survivors using anti-Mullerian hormone. Hum Reprod. 2009;24(4):982–90.
34. Wong QHY, Anderson RA. The role of antimullerian hormone in assessing ovarian damage from chemotherapy, radiotherapy and surgery. Curr Opin Endocrinol Diabetes Obes. 2018;25(6):391–8.
35. Kim HA, Choi J, Park CS, Seong MK, Hong SE, Kim JS, et al. Post-chemotherapy serum anti-Mullerian hormone level predicts ovarian function recovery. Endocr Connect. 2018;7(8):949–56.
36. Reifschneider K, Auble BA, Rose SR. Update of endocrine dysfunction following pediatric traumatic brain injury. J Clin Med. 2015;4(8):1536–60.
37. Deligeoroglou E, Athanasopoulos N, Tsimaris P, Dimopoulos KD, Vrachnis N, Creatsas G. Evaluation and management of adolescent amenorrhea. Ann NY Acad Sci. 2010;1205:23–32.
38. Passos I, Britto RL. Diagnosis and treatment of mullerian malformations. Taiwan J Obstet Gynecol. 2020;59(2):183–8.
39. Kapczuk K, Kedzia W. Primary amenorrhea due to anatomical abnormalities of the reproductive tract: molecular insight. Int J Mol Sci. 2021;22(21):11495.
40. Sultan C, Biason-Lauber A, Philibert P. Mayer-Rokitansky-Kuster-Hauser syndrome: recent clinical and genetic findings. Gynecol Endocrinol. 2009;25(1):8–11.
41. Patel S, Zhou C, Rattan S, Flaws JA. Effects of endocrine-disrupting chemicals on the ovary. Biol Reprod. 2015;93(1):20.
42. Vabre P, Gatimel N, Moreau J, Gayrard V, Picard-Hagen N, Parinaud J, et al. Environmental pollutants, a possible etiology for premature ovarian insufficiency: a narrative review of animal and human data. Environ Health. 2017;16(1):37.
43. Gigante E, Picciocchi E, Valenzano A, Dell'Orco S. The effects of the endocrine disruptors and of the halogens on the female reproductive system and on epigenetics: a brief review. Acta Med Mediterr. 2018;34:1295.
44. Seppa S, Kuiri-Hanninen T, Holopainen E, Voutilainen R. MANAGEMENT OF ENDOCRINE DISEASE: diagnosis and management of primary amenorrhea and female delayed puberty. Eur J Endocrinol. 2021;184(6):R225–R42.
45. Kaldewey SKL. Different approaches to Hormone Replacement Therapy in women with premature ovarian insufficiency. Gynecol Reprod Endocrinol Metab. 2021;2(3):134–9.
46. Huhtaniemi I, Hovatta O, La Marca A, Livera G, Monniaux D, Persani L, et al. Advances in the molecular pathophysiology, genetics, and treatment of primary ovarian insufficiency. Trends Endocrinol Metab. 2018;29(6):400–19.
47. Jung EJ, Im DH, Park YH, Byun JM, Kim YN, Jeong DH, et al. Female with 46, XY karyotype. Obstet Gynecol Sci. 2017;60(4):378–82.

Amenorrhea in Eating Disorders

Angelica Lindén Hirschberg

3.1   Introduction

Eating disorders are one of the leading causes of disease burden through disability or death for young women during their reproductive years. They include anorexia nervosa (AN), bulimia nervosa (BN), binge eating disorder, avoidant-restrictive food intake disorder, pica, and rumination disorder. However, the two main diagnoses are AN, characterized by severe underweight, intense fear of becoming fat, and disturbed body perception, and BN with typical symptoms of recurrent episodes of binge eating in combination with inappropriate compensatory behavior like self-induced vomiting. Both AN and BN are associated with endocrinological abnormalities, which can lead to amenorrhea. However, there are various underlying causes of amenorrhea in women with eating disorders. This chapter addresses mechanisms and contributing factors to amenorrhea in AN and BN, long-term medical consequences, and management of amenorrhea in women with eating disorders.

3.2   Anorexia Nervosa

AN is a serious psychiatric illness that mainly affects adolescent girls and young women with distorted body image and who engage in excessive dieting leading to severe weight loss and a pathological fear of becoming fat [1]. Diagnostic criteria of AN according to DSM-V [2] are shown in Table 3.1. AN has two subtypes: AN restricting type, characterized by restriction of food intake without binging or

A. L. Hirschberg (✉)
Department of Women's and Children's Health, Karolinska Institutet, Solna, Sweden

Department of Gynecology and Reproductive Medicine, Karolinska University Hospital, Stockholm, Sweden
e-mail: angelica.linden-hirschberg@sll.se

© International Society of Gynecological Endocrinology 2023
A. R. Genazzani et al. (eds.), *Amenorrhea*, ISGE Series,
https://doi.org/10.1007/978-3-031-22378-5_3

Table 3.1 Diagnostic criteria of anorexia nervosa according to DSM-V [1]

(A)	Restriction of energy intake relative to requirements, leading to a significantly low body weight in the context of age, sex, developmental trajectory, and physical health. Significantly low weight is defined as a weight that is less than minimally normal or, for children and adolescents, less than minimally expected
(B)	Intense fear of gaining weight or of becoming fat, or persistent behavior that interferes with weight gain, even though at a significantly low weight
(C)	Disturbance in the way in which one's body weight or shape is experienced, undue influence of body weight or shape on self-evaluation, or persistent lack of recognition of the seriousness of the current low body weight

Restrictive type: During the last 3 months, the individual has not engaged in recurrent episodes of binge eating or purging behavior (i.e., self-induced vomiting, or misuse of laxatives, diuretics, or enemas). This subtype describes presentations in which weight loss is accomplished primarily through dieting, fasting, and/or excessive exercise

Binge eating/purging type: During the last 3 months, the individual has engaged in recurrent episodes of binge eating or purging behavior (i.e., self-induced vomiting, or misuse of laxatives, diuretics, or enemas)

Current severity:
Mild: BMI more than 17
Moderate: BMI between 16 and 16.99
Severe: BMI between 15 and 15.99
Extreme: BMI less than 15

purging, and AN binge eating/purging type, in which individuals engage in binge eating followed by compensatory behaviors like self-induced vomiting or misuse of laxatives [2]. The previous DSM-IV criterion amenorrhea has been deleted since the criterion cannot be applied to males, premenarcheal females, females taking oral contraceptives, and postmenopausal women [3]. Still, amenorrhea is a characteristic feature of AN.

The lifetime prevalence of AN in women has been estimated between 1 and 4% depending on the criteria used, and for men it is about ten times less prevalent [4]. The overall incidence rate of AN has been stable over the past decades, but there has been an increase in the high-risk group of 15–19-year-old girls [1]. Long-term follow-up studies (>20 years) have shown that about a third of the patients have a persistent eating disorder [5], and the mortality rate is severely increased with a standardized mortality rate of 5.9 [6]. In addition to consequences of starvation, suicide is a common cause of death in AN [6].

The etiology of AN remains incompletely understood. Typical personality features of individuals with AN include perfectionism, compulsivity, anxiety, harm avoidance, and low self-esteem [1]. The most common comorbid psychiatric conditions include major depression and anxiety disorder [7]. Other risk factors are genetic predisposition, social isolation, and psychosocial stress [1]. Furthermore, disturbances in neurotransmitter systems including serotonin and dopamine have been implicated in the disorder [8]. The ultimate understanding of AN etiology will likely include the main effects of genetic, biological, and environmental factors, as well as their interactions and correlations.

3.2.1   Physical Signs of AN

The most obvious sign of AN is severe underweight (Fig. 3.1). Medical complications of AN affect all organ systems and are primarily consequences of starvation, malnutrition, and purging [1]. They include the cardiovascular system with symptoms of hypotension, bradycardia, arrhythmias, and hypovolemia, as well as electrolyte disturbances leading to sodium depletion, hypophosphatemia, and hypomagnesemia. Gastrointestinal symptoms with nausea and constipation are common and bothersome. Dental problems can be due to reduced saliva production and self-induced vomiting. Cognitive and emotional functioning is markedly disturbed. AN is also associated with extensive endocrine abnormalities leading to symptoms of hypometabolism including low body temp, dry skin, cold hands and feet, arrested growth, and loss of bone mass, as well as reproductive failure with delay in puberty development and amenorrhea.

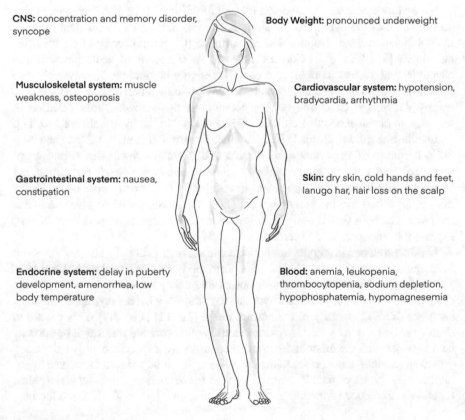

Anorexia nervosa

CNS: concentration and memory disorder, syncope

Body Weight: pronounced underweight

Musculoskeletal system: muscle weakness, osteoporosis

Cardiovascular system: hypotension, bradycardia, arrhythmia

Gastrointestinal system: nausea, constipation

Skin: dry skin, cold hands and feet, lanugo har, hair loss on the scalp

Endocrine system: delay in puberty development, amenorrhea, low body temperature

Blood: anemia, leukopenia, thrombocytopenia, sodium depletion, hypophosphatemia, hypomagnesemia

Fig. 3.1 Physical symptoms in women with AN

3.3   Functional Hypothalamic Amenorrhea

AN can be associated with both primary amenorrhea (spontaneous menstruation has never occurred) or secondary amenorrhea (absence of menstruation for at least three consecutive months) and occasionally oligomenorrhea meaning menstruation at increased intervals (>6 weeks, 5–9 periods during the past year).

3.3.1   Endocrine Disturbances

Amenorrhea in AN is attributed to a functional inhibition of the hypothalamic-pituitary-gonadal (HPG) axis, i.e., functional hypothalamic amenorrhea (FHA) caused by low energy availability and undernutrition often in combination with excessive physical exercise [9, 10]. This leads to a disruption of the pulsatile release of gonadotropin-releasing hormone (GnRH), which in turn causes a reduced secretion of luteinizing hormone (LH) and follicle-stimulating hormone (FSH) from the pituitary resulting in attenuated ovarian production of estradiol, progesterone, and testosterone and subsequent anovulation and amenorrhea (Fig. 3.2).

Several mechanisms are involved in such inhibition of the HPG axis, including an activation of the hypothalamic-pituitary-adrenal axis and a consequent increase in hypothalamic corticotropin-releasing hormone (CRH) and cortisol from the adrenal glands [11] (Fig. 3.2). Cortisol increases in situations of acute physical and psychological distress to mobilize glucose for energy production. However, chronic elevation of cortisol levels at rest indicates catabolic metabolism and adaptation to energy deficiency. CRH and cortisol together with the endorphins, released in response to physical activity, inhibit GnRH secretion in the hypothalamus [10, 11].

Insulin-like growth factor I (IGF-I), which is secreted from the liver, is an anabolic hormone of importance for muscle and skeletal growth and a peripheral marker of nutritional status. Secondary to chronic energy deficiency and circulating levels of insulin and IGF-I are reduced, and levels of growth hormone and IGF-binding protein-1 are increased [10, 11] (Fig. 3.2). Because IGF-I also stimulates the release of both GnRH and LH, a decline in IGF-I activity may, at least in part, explain the reduction in LH secretion.

Leptin, produced in adipocytes, is also a marker of nutritional status and involved in the pulsatile secretion of GnRH. This hormone is markedly reduced in AN [10–12] (Fig. 3.2). Furthermore, thyroid hormones, and particularly triiodothyronine (T3), are reduced in response to a hypometabolic state, whereas thyroid-stimulating hormone (TSH) is usually in the normal range [10, 11] (Fig. 3.2). This condition should not be treated by levothyroxine since thyroid hormone status will be normalized together with the other endocrine disturbances by improved energy balance.

Taken together, amenorrhea related to AN can be explained by a functional hypothalamic inhibition of the reproductive system by stress hormones and endorphins, together with reduced stimulation of GnRH due to low levels of IGF-I and leptin.

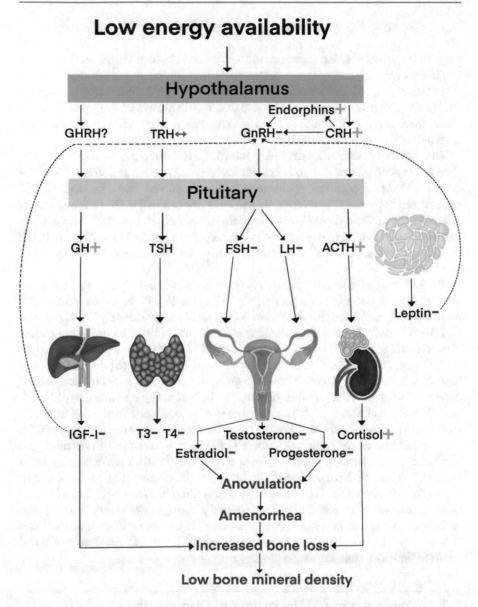

Fig. 3.2 A summary of endocrine disturbances associated with functional hypothalamic amenorrhea in AN. + indicates increased levels, − indicates reduced levels. *ACTH* adrenocorticotropic hormone, *CRH* corticotrophin-releasing hormone, *FSH* follicle-stimulating hormone, *GH* growth hormone, *GHRH* growth hormone-releasing hormone, *GnRH* gonadotropin-releasing hormone, *IGF-I* insulin-like growth factor-I, *LH* luteinizing hormone

3.4   Medical Consequences of Hypothalamic Amenorrhea

In young individuals, the endocrine disturbances related to FHA and AN often result in delayed puberty development including inhibited growth and primary amenorrhea [13, 14]. Definitions of delayed puberty in girls are no pubertal signs by age 13 or no menstruation by age 16, and this should always be evaluated. In these cases, there is a risk of failure to reach peak bone mass, as well as to obtain lower final height than expected [13, 14].

One obvious consequence of FHA is infertility. However, hypothalamic amenorrhea is a functional disorder and does not involve any organic pathology. Such disorders can be normalized spontaneously by improved nutrition and weight restoration. For those who recover, infertility is rarely a major clinical problem. In other cases, the focus should be on the treatment of AN. Women with eating disorders have an increased risk of adverse pregnancy and neonatal outcomes [15, 16]. It is therefore not appropriate to promote fertility treatment in these women before recovery.

FHA is associated with a rapid loss of bone mass, particularly of trabecular bone such as the lumbar spine and pelvis (Fig. 3.2) [17, 18]. If the condition remains untreated, it is estimated that the loss of bone mass is approximately 2–3% per year and there is risk of irreversible changes of bone mass [19]. The definition of low bone mineral density (BMD) in a premenopausal woman is a Z-score (i.e., standard deviation score of the mean of an age- and sex-matched reference population) lower than 2, whereas osteoporosis in this age group is defined as a Z-score less than 2 combined with secondary clinical risk factors such as eating disorders, hypogonadism, or previous fracture [20]. The prevalence of osteoporosis in girls/women with AN is 50% [21]. Furthermore, the risk of stress fracture is several times increased [22].

The mechanisms of bone loss involve both suppression of bone formation and increased bone resorption caused by the combination of nutritional deficiency and a catabolic hormone balance including estrogen deficiency (Fig. 3.2) [23, 24]. Estrogen is important for bone turnover and acts through specific receptors in bone tissue to prevent bone resorption. Consequently, estrogen deficiency is associated with bone loss due to increased bone resorption [23]. Chronic elevation of cortisol can also contribute to increased bone resorption [25], whereas low levels of IGF-I result in impaired bone formation [24].

3.5   Management of Hypothalamic Amenorrhea

Amenorrhea should always be evaluated although this is an expected finding in girls/women with AN. Gynecological examination is not always necessary and especially not if the individual is adolescent or virgin. However, endocrinological evaluation should be performed to confirm the underlying cause of amenorrhea. FHA is characterized by clearly suppressed levels of LH and low levels of FSH, estradiol, testosterone, and T3, whereas levels of sex hormone-binding globulin (SHBG) are elevated (Table 3.2) [10, 26, 27]. When evaluating FHA, laboratory

Table 3.2 Typical endocrine findings in functional hypothalamic amenorrhea (FHA) and polycystic ovary syndrome (PCOS)

Hormone or binding protein	FHA	PCOS
FSH	↓	↔
LH	↓↓	↑
Estradiol	↓	↔
Testosterone	↓	↑
SHBG	↑	↓
Prolactin	↓	↔
TSH	↔	↔ ↑
Free T4/T3	↓	↔ ↓

FSH follicle-stimulating hormone, LH luteinizing hormone, SHBG sex hormone-binding globulin, TSH thyroid-stimulating hormone, T4 thyroxine, T3 triiodothyronine

tests should also include measurement of complete blood count, electrolytes and liver panel, and other relevant nutritional factors [27].

Since long-standing FHA and low energy availability are associated with a loss of bone mass and increased risk of musculoskeletal injuries, bone mass should be assessed in adult patients preferably by dual-energy X-ray absorptiometry (DXA), which is the golden standard method for assessment of bone mass and body composition including body fat [27].

FHA is an acquired condition that can be normalized once the energy balance has been restored. Correcting energy balance including increased caloric intake and/or decreased exercise activity should therefore always be the first-line strategy of intervention in women with FHA, and counseling by a dietitian or nutritionist is recommended besides specific treatment of AN [27]. Optimized energy intake and increased body weight/fat mass have documented effect on restoration of menstrual function in women with FHA [28]. In case of low bone mass, supplementation of calcium and vitamin D may also be beneficial.

One year without resumption of menses should lead to consideration of pharmacological treatment particularly in patients with severe bone loss (osteoporosis) or fracture history. Bisphosphonates are not recommended since this treatment is not approved for use in premenopausal women. Transdermal estrogen in combination

Table 3.3 Take-home message of amenorrhea in women with anorexia nervosa (AN)

• Hormonal disturbances are primarily secondary to starvation leading to functional hypothalamic amenorrhea (FHA)
• Long-standing FHA and inhibited pubertal development in AN adversely affect bone mass
• Recommendation against oral contraceptives for the purpose of regaining menses or improving bone mass
• Recommendation against bisphosphonates for improvement of bone mass
• Increased caloric intake and/or decreased exercise activity should always be the first-line strategy to restore menstrual function in women with FHA
• Short-term use of transdermal estradiol with cyclic progesterone/progestogen could be considered in patients with chronic disease

with cyclic progesterone/progestogen could be considered. This treatment has been demonstrated to improve bone mass in adolescent girls with AN [29]. However, oral estrogen like in oral contraceptives should be avoided since oral estrogen has a suppressive effect on hepatic IGF-I [30], which is a bone trophic factor [24]. It should be noted that low BMD is not the only indication for estrogen substitution in women with FHA but also a treatment of other symptoms of estrogen deficiency such as endothelial dysfunction, adverse lipid profile, urogenital symptoms, dyspareunia, and sexual dysfunction [27]. Take-home message for amenorrhea in women with AN is presented in Table 3.3.

3.6   Treatment of AN

The treatment of AN aims at restoring weight; normalizing eating behavior; treating psychological disturbances such as distortion of body image, low self-esteem, and interpersonal conflicts; and achieving long-term remission and rehabilitation, and eventually full recovery [1]. In the acute phase of malnutrition and severe weight loss, hospitalization is needed for refeeding and medical stabilization. In the outpatient treatment of AN, there is evidence for family-based therapy in young individuals [31, 32]. In adults, different types of outpatient psychotherapy such as specialist supportive clinical management, cognitive behavioral therapy (CBT), and interpersonal psychotherapy have demonstrated similar results [33–35]. Approximately, 25% of patients recover completely, and 25% fail to respond to the treatment. Pharmacotherapy with antidepressants may be a complement but is not recommended as a single treatment [1].

3.7   Bulimia Nervosa

BN is a mental disorder characterized by self-perpetuating and self-defeating cycles of binge eating and regular use of inappropriate compensatory behavior in order to prevent weight gain [1]. During a "binge," the person consumes a large amount of food in a rapid, automatic, and uncontrolled fashion. This may anesthetize hunger,

Table 3.4 Diagnostic criteria of bulimia nervosa according to DSM-V [1]

(A)	Recurrent episodes of binge eating characterized by both:
	1. Eating in a discrete period of time, an amount of food that is definitely larger than what most individuals would eat in a similar period of time under similar circumstances
	2. A sense of lack of control over eating during the episodes
(B)	Recurrent inappropriate compensatory behaviors to prevent weight gain, such as self-induced vomiting; misuse of laxatives, diuretics, or other medications; fasting; or excessive exercise
(C)	The binge eating and inappropriate compensatory behaviors both occur, on average, at least once a week for 3 months
(D)	Self-evaluation is unduly influenced by body shape and weight
(E)	The disturbance does not occur exclusively during episodes of anorexia nervosa

Current severity:
Mild: An average of 1–3 episodes of inappropriate compensatory behaviors per week
Moderate: An average of 4–7 episodes of inappropriate compensatory behaviors per week
Severe: An average of 8–13 episodes of inappropriate compensatory behaviors per week
Extreme: An average of 14 or more episodes of inappropriate compensatory behaviors per week

tension, anger, and other feelings, but it eventually creates physical discomfort and anxiety about weight gain. Thus, the person "purges" the food eaten, usually by inducing vomiting or by misuse of laxatives and diuretics. The individual may also resort to other compensatory behaviors, such as restrictive dieting and excessive exercise. Diagnostic criteria of BN according to DSM-V are presented in Table 3.4 [2]. Compared to the previous DSM-IV criteria, the frequency of binge eating and compensatory behaviors that individuals with BN must exhibit has been reduced from twice weekly to once a week.

The lifetime prevalence rate of BN is around 2% in young females [4]. Unfortunately, because of the denial, embarrassment, shame, and secrecy associated with bulimia, the illness can often go unacknowledged, delaying assessment and intervention. The reported prevalence rate of BN can therefore only serve as a minimum estimate of the true prevalence. The peak age of incidence of BN is 16–20 years of age and thus later than in AN. However, several studies suggest that age at onset of BN is decreasing [1]. Little is known about the long-term course and outcome of BN. However, available data indicate remission rates up to 70% or more by 10-year follow-up of BN [36]. BN is associated with lower mortality rates than AN. In a meta-analysis, the overall standardized mortality ratio for BN was 1.9 [6].

The etiology of bulimia is unknown but genetic, biological, social, and psychological factors all seem to play a role [1]. Familial factors increase the risk of developing the disorder, and twin studies reveal a moderate to substantial contribution of additive genetic factors [37]. Comorbidity is also common, and about 50% of women with BN have symptoms of attention deficit hyperactivity disorder (ADHD), atypical depression, and anxiety [1]. Furthermore, BN is associated with borderline personality disorder, substance abuse, and compulsive disorders [1]. Serotonergic function has also been implicated in BN [38].

3.7.1   Physical Signs of BN

BN is not typically associated with the serious physical complications normally associated with AN, mainly because most women with BN are of normal weight (Fig. 3.3). However, commonly they report physical symptoms such as fatigue, lethargy, bloating, and gastrointestinal problems [1]. Individuals with BN who engage in frequent vomiting may experience electrolyte abnormalities, metabolic alkalosis, esophageal irritation, chest pain, erosion of dental enamel, swelling of parotid glands, and scars and calluses on the backs of their hands [1]. Those who frequently misuse laxatives can have edema, fluid loss and subsequent dehydration, electrolyte abnormalities, metabolic acidosis, and potentially permanent loss of normal bowel function [1]. BN is also associated with endocrine and reproductive disorders including amenorrhea/oligomenorrhea although most women with BN are not underweight.

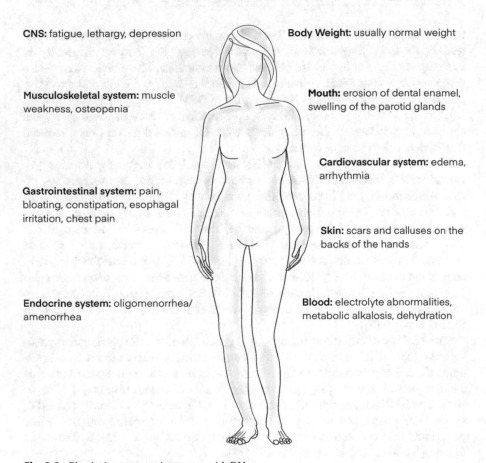

Bulimia nervosa

CNS: fatigue, lethargy, depression

Body Weight: usually normal weight

Musculoskeletal system: muscle weakness, osteopenia

Mouth: erosion of dental enamel, swelling of the parotid glands

Cardiovascular system: edema, arrhythmia

Gastrointestinal system: pain, bloating, constipation, esophagal irritation, chest pain

Skin: scars and calluses on the backs of the hands

Endocrine system: oligomenorrhea/amenorrhea

Blood: electrolyte abnormalities, metabolic alkalosis, dehydration

Fig. 3.3 Physical symptoms in women with BN

3.8   Menstrual Disturbances in BN

The occurrence of amenorrhea in bulimic women has been reported within the range of 7–40%, and 37–64% of patients may have irregular bleedings with long intervals (oligomenorrhea) [39]. In comparison, the prevalence of secondary amenorrhea in the general population is between 2 and 5% [40].

Different mechanisms may interact in the etiology of amenorrhea/oligomenorrhea in BN. In AN, amenorrhea is explained by FHA, i.e., hypothalamic inhibition of the reproductive system due to starvation [9, 10]. Low levels of estradiol and gonadotropins, indicating hypothalamic inhibition of the HPG axis [41], as well as low levels of thyroid hormones, have also been reported in bulimic women [42, 43]. These endocrine disturbances are considered to be related to temporary starvation and large weight changes in women with BN.

In addition, an association between bulimia and polycystic ovary syndrome (PCOS) has been suggested [39, 44]. PCOS is the most common hormonal aberration in women of fertile age, with a prevalence of 10%, and is associated with oligomenorrhea/amenorrhea due to oligo- or anovulation, clinical symptoms of hyperandrogenism (hirsutism and acne), and polycystic ovaries on ultrasound [45]. Diagnostic criteria for PCOS are presented in Table 3.5 [46]. Furthermore, the syndrome is often associated with insulin resistance and abdominal obesity. The etiology of PCOS is still largely unknown, but there is strong evidence for a genetic predisposition, although environmental factors also play a part [45].

Table 3.5 The diagnostic criteria for PCOS according to Rotterdam Consensus 2004 [46]

Diagnostic criteria for PCOS
1. Oligo- or anovulation
2. Clinical and/or biochemical signs of hyperandrogenism
3. Polycystic ovaries on ultrasound

Two out of three criteria are necessary for diagnosis

3.9   Association Between Bulimia and PCOS

There are several similarities between PCOS and BN. Disturbed appetite regulation, increased craving for carbohydrates, and an increased prevalence of eating disorders have been reported in women with PCOS [47, 48]. On the other hand, an increased frequency of PCOS symptoms has been demonstrated in bulimic women in comparison with healthy controls. Thus, increased occurrence of polycystic ovaries, acne, and hirsutism and elevated serum levels of androgens have been reported in bulimic women [49–51].

What is the etiological connection between bulimia and PCOS? It has been suggested that polycystic ovaries may be secondary to abnormal eating behavior [50]. Another explanation for an association between bulimia and PCOS may be that hyperandrogenism is the primary condition, which predisposes for the development of bulimic behavior and associated psychiatric comorbidity. Testosterone is appetite stimulating [44], and high androgen levels in women have been associated with impaired impulse control, irritability, anxiety, and depression [52, 53]. These symptoms are common features in women with bulimia [52]. Furthermore, bulimic women are more sexually experienced and sexually experimental than control women [54]. This may also be related to increased androgen activity since androgens have well-known stimulatory effects on female sexuality [55].

It could be concluded that BN is associated with several hormonal aberrations, which may be primary or secondary to abnormal eating. Menstrual disturbances may be caused by hypothalamic inhibition of the reproductive axis due to periods of starvation. An alternative explanation is essential hyperandrogenism like PCOS, which may promote bulimic behavior since androgens have appetite-stimulating effects and could impair impulse control.

3.9.1   Antiandrogenic Treatment

It was suggested that treatment with antiandrogenic activity may be effective as an additional therapy for bulimic women. In support of this hypothesis, the androgen receptor antagonist flutamide has been shown to reduce symptoms in bulimic patients [56]. However, this medication is associated with adverse liver effects, which would limit the long-term use of the drug. It was also demonstrated that treatment with an antiandrogenic combined oral contraceptive (30 μg ethinylestradiol + 3 mg drospirenone) improved eating behavior and reduced meal-related appetite in relation to decreased testosterone levels by the treatment in women with BN [57]. The results support the notion that androgens play a role in bulimic behavior. Hypothetically, BN may in some cases be a manifestation of a hormonal constitution rather than a primary psychiatric illness.

3.10 Management of Amenorrhea in BN

The two most common underlying mechanisms to oligomenorrhea/amenorrhea in women with BN seem to be FHA and PCOS. Endocrine evaluation should always be performed for proper management according to the underlying cause. It has already been mentioned above that the typical endocrine findings in FHA are low levels of gonadotropins, estradiol, and thyroid hormones but high levels of SHBG, whereas PCOS is associated with increased LH/FSH ratio, high levels of testosterone, and low levels of SHBG (Table 3.2). In most cases, there is an obvious difference in the hormonal profile between FHA and PCOS (Table 3.2); however, in some women with BN, it can be a mixed picture of both FHA and PCOS.

Bulimic women may have low bone mass secondary to FHA, particularly those with previous AN [43, 58]. DXA should therefore be performed in those women. In PCOS, hyperandrogenism appears to provide good protection from bone loss despite oligomenorrhea/amenorrhea in women with BN [10].

It is recommended that FHA in women with BN is managed as in AN; see above and Table 3.3. In bulimic women with PCOS, antiandrogenic oral contraceptives could be considered. Combined oral contraceptives regulate menstruations, improve symptoms of hirsutism and acne, and may improve bulimic symptoms by antiandrogenic effects [57]. Take-home message for amenorrhea in women with BN is presented in Table 3.6.

Table 3.6 Take-home message of amenorrhea/oligomenorrhea in women with bulimia nervosa (BN)

• Menstrual disorders are common in BN despite normal body weight
• Both functional hypothalamic amenorrhea (FHA) and polycystic ovary syndrome (PCOS) are associated with BN
• Menstrual disorders should always be investigated by endocrine evaluation for proper management according to the underlying cause
• FHA in women with BN should be managed as in anorexia nervosa; see Table 3.2
• In those with PCOS, antiandrogenic oral contraceptives may be a complement to conventional therapy for treatment of BN

3.11 Treatment of BN

The primary goal of treatment for bulimia is to reduce or eliminate binge eating and purging behavior [1]. In adolescents, family-based therapy is one of the first-line treatment recommendations [59]. In adults, CBT is the recommended state-of-the-art treatment [59]. Furthermore, nutritional rehabilitation and psychosocial intervention are often employed. Establishment of a pattern of regular, non-binge meals, improvement of attitudes related to eating, encouragement of healthy but not excessive exercise, and resolution of co-occurring conditions such as mood or anxiety disorders are among the specific aims of these strategies [59]. In addition to psychotherapy, medical treatment can be necessary in many cases. Fluoxetine is the medication of choice; however, a meta-analysis revealed that fluoxetine had negligible efficacy in promoting remission [60].

3.12 Conclusion

In conclusion, AN and BN are both associated with amenorrhea, which should always be investigated by endocrine evaluation for proper management according to diagnosis. The underlying cause of amenorrhea in AN is usually a consequence of starvation and underweight leading to a functional inhibition of the HPG axis (FHA) resulting in suppressed levels of gonadotropins and estradiol. Puberty development may be negatively affected, and there is an increased risk of bone loss. BN, on the other hand, is associated with PCOS and increased androgen levels, which hypothetically may promote bulimic behavior by influencing food craving or impulse control. As in AN, BN is also associated with FHA probably due to temporary starvation although body weight is normal. FHA can be normalized once energy balance is restored. However, in the absence of recovery by psychotherapy and nutritional counseling, substitution with transdermal estrogen could be considered. In those with PCOS, antiandrogenic oral contraceptives may be a complement to conventional therapy for treatment of BN.

References

1. Treasure J, Duarte TA, Schmidt U. Eating disorders. Lancet. 2020;395:899–911.
2. American Psychiatric Association. Diagnostic and statistical manual of mental disorders. 5th ed. Washington, DC: American Psychiatric Press; 2013.
3. Mustelin L, Silén Y, Raevuori A, Hoek HW, Kaprio J, Keski-Rahkonen A. The DSM-5 diagnostic criteria for anorexia nervosa may change its population prevalence and prognostic value. J Psychiatry Res. 2016;77:85–91.
4. Smink FRE, van Hoeken D, Hoek HW. Epidemiology, course, and outcome of eating disorders. Curr Opin Psychiatry. 2013;26(6):543–8.
5. Dobrescu SR, Dinkler L, Gillberg C, Råstam M, Gillberg C, Wentz E. Anorexia nervosa: 30-year outcome. Br J Psychiatry. 2019;22:1–8.
6. Arcelus J, Mitchell AJ, Wales J, Nielsen S. Mortality rates in patients with anorexia nervosa and other eating disorders. A meta-analysis of 36 studies. Arch Gen Psychiatry. 2011;68:724–31.

7. Marucci S, Ragione LD, DeIaco G, Mococci T, Vicini M, Guastamacchia E, Triggiani V. Anorexia nervosa and comorbid psychopathology. Endocr Metab Immune Disord Drug Targets. 2018;18(4):316–24.
8. Riva G. Neurobiology of anorexia nervosa: serotonin dysfunctions link self-starvation with body image disturbances through an impaired body memory. Front Hum Neurosci. 2016;10:600.
9. Allaway HCM, Southmayd EA, De Souza MJ. The physiology of functional hypothalamic amenorrhea associated with energy deficiency in exercising women and in women with anorexia nervosa. Horm Mol Biol Clin Investig. 2016;25(2):91–119.
10. Hirschberg AL. Female hyperandrogenism and elite sport. Endocr Connect. 2020;9:R81–92.
11. Misra M, Klibanski A. Endocrine consequences of anorexia nervosa. Lancet Diabetes Endocrinol. 2014;2:581–92.
12. Müller TD, Föcker M, Holtkamp K, Herpertz-Dahlmann B, Hebebrand J. Leptin-mediated neuroendocrine alterations in anorexia nervosa: somatic and behavioral implications. Child Adolesc Psychiatr Clin N Am. 2009;18(1):117–29.
13. Muñoz-Calvo MT, Argente J. Nutritional and pubertal disorders. Endocr Dev. 2016;29:153–73.
14. Neale J, Pais SMA, Nicholls D, Chapman S, Hudson LD. What are the effects of restrictive eating disorders on growth and puberty and are effects permanent? A systematic review and meta-analysis. J Adolesc Health. 2020;66(2):144–56.
15. Kouba S, Lindholm C, Hällström T, Hirschberg AL. Pregnancy and neonatal outcomes in women with eating disorders—a prospective controlled study. Obstet Gynecol. 2005;105:255–60.
16. Mantel Ä, Hirschberg AL, Stephansson O. Association of maternal eating disorders with pregnancy and neonatal outcomes. JAMA Psychiatry. 2020;77(3):285–93.
17. Shufelt CL, Torbati T, Dutra E. Hypothalamic amenorrhea and the long-term health consequences. Semin Reprod Med. 2017;35:256–62.
18. Misra M, Klibanski A. Bone metabolism in adolescents with anorexia nervosa. J Endocrinol Investig. 2011;34(4):324–32.
19. Miller KK, Lee EE, Lawson EA, Misra M, Minihan J, Grinspoon SK, Gleysteen S, Mickley D, Herzog D, Klibanski A. Determinants of skeletal loss and recovery in anorexia nervosa. J Clin Endocrinol Metab. 2006;91:2931–7.
20. Lewiecki EM, Gordon CM, Baim S, Leonard MB, Bishop NJ, Bianchi M-L, Kalkwarf HJ, Langman CB, Plotkin H, Rauch F, Zemel BS, Binkley N, Bilezikian JP, Kendler DL, Hans DB, Silverman S. International Society for Clinical Densitometry 2007 adult and Pediatric Official Positions. Bone. 2008;43:1115–21.
21. Legroux-Gerot I, Vignau J, Collier F, Cortet B. Bone loss associated with anorexia nervosa. Joint Bone Spine. 2005;72:489–95.
22. Faje AT, Fazeli PK, Miller KK, Katzman DK, Ebrahimi S, Lee H, Mendes N, Snelgrove D, Meenaghan E, Misra M, Klibanski A. Fracture risk and areal bone mineral density in adolescent females with anorexia nervosa. Int J Eat Disord. 2014;47(5):458–66.
23. Almeida M, Laurent MR, Dubois V, Claessens F, O'Brien CA, Bouillon R, Vanderschueren D, Manolagas SC. Estrogens and androgens in skeletal physiology and pathophysiology. Physiol Rev. 2017;97:135–87.
24. Snow CM, Rosen CJ, Robinson TL. Serum IGF-I is higher in gymnasts than runners and predicts bone and lean mass. Med Sci Sports Exerc. 2000;32:1902–7.
25. Tauchmanovà L, Pivonello R, De Martino MC, Rusciano A, De Leo M, Ruosi C, Mainolfi C, Lombardi G, Salvatore M, Colao A. Effects of sex steroids on bone in women with subclinical or overt endogenous hypercortisolism. Eur J Endocrinol. 2007;157:359–66.
26. Rickenlund A, Thorén M, Carlström K, von Schoultz B, Hirschberg AL. Diurnal profiles of testosterone and pituitary hormones suggest different mechanisms for menstrual disturbances in endurance athletes. J Clin Endocrinol Metab. 2004;89:702–7.
27. Gordon CM, Ackerman KE, Berga SL, Kaplan JR, Mastorakos G, Misra M, Murad MH, Santoro NF, Warren MP. Functional hypothalamic amenorrhea: an Endocrine Society clinical practice guideline. J Clin Endocrinol Metab. 2017;102:1413–39.

28. Misra M, Prabhakaran R, Miller KK, Goldstein MA, Mickley D, Clauss L, Lockhart P, Cord J, Herzog DB, Katzman DK, Klibanski A. Weight gain and restoration of menses as predictors of bone mineral density change in adolescent girls with anorexia nervosa-1. J Clin Endocrinol Metab. 2008;93:1231–7.

29. Misra M, Katzman D, Miller KK, Mendes N, Snelgrove D, Russell M, Goldstein MA, Ebrahimi S, Clauss L, Weigel T, Mickley D, Schoenfeld DA, Herzog DB, Klibanski A. Physiologic estrogen replacement increases bone density in adolescent girls with anorexia nervosa. J Bone Miner Res. 2011;26:2430–8.

30. Weissberger AJ, Ho KK, Lazarus L. Contrasting effects of oral and transdermal routes of estrogen replacement therapy on 24-hour growth hormone (GH) secretion, insulin-like growth factor I, and GH-binding protein in postmenopausal women. J Clin Endocrinol Metab. 1991;72(2):374–81.

31. Hilbert A, Hoek HW, Schmidt R. Evidence-based clinical guidelines for eating disorders: international comparison. Curr Opin Psychiatry. 2017;30:423–37.

32. Fisher CA, Skocic S, Rutherford KA, Hetrick SE. Family therapy approaches for anorexia nervosa. Cochrane Database Syst Rev. 2019. Published online May 1. https://doi.org/10.1002/14651858.CD004780.pub4.

33. van den Berg E, Houtzager L, de Vos J, Daemen I, Katsaragaki G, Karyotaki E, Cuijpers P, Dekker J. Meta-analysis on the efficacy of psychological treatments for anorexia nervosa. Eur Eat Disord Rev. 2019;27:331–51.

34. Zeeck A, Herpertz-Dahlmann B, Friederich HC, Brockmeyer T, Resmark G, Hagenah U, Ehrlich S, Cuntz U, Zipfel S, Hartmann A. Psychotherapeutic treatment for anorexia nervosa: a systematic review and network meta-analysis. Front Psychiatry. 2018;9:158.

35. Hay PJ, Touyz S, Claudino AM, Lujic S, Smith CA, Madden S. Inpatient versus outpatient care, partial hospitalisation and waiting list for people with eating disorders. Cochrane Database Syst Rev. 2019;1:CD010827.

36. Keel PK, Brown TA. Update on course and outcome in eating disorders. Int J Eat Disord. 2010;43:195–204.

37. Carter FA, McIntosh VV, Joyce PR, Frampton CM, Bulik CM. Bulimia nervosa, childbirth, and psychopathology. J Psychosom Res. 2003;55:357–61.

38. Steiger H, Bruce KR, Groleau P. Neural circuits, neurotransmitters, and behavior: serotonin and temperament in bulimic syndromes. Curr Top Behav Neurosci. 2011;6:125–38.

39. Kimmel MC, Ferguson EH, Zerwas S, Bulik CM, Meltzer-Brody S. Obstetric and gynecologic problems associated with eating disorders. Int J Eat Disord. 2016;49(3):260–75.

40. Münster K, Helm P, Schmidt L. Secondary amenorrhoea: prevalence and medical contact—a cross–sectional study from a Danish county. Br J Obstet Gynaecol. 1992;99:430–3.

41. Resch M, Szendei G, Haász P. Eating disorders from a gynecologic and endocrinologic view: hormonal changes. Fertil Steril. 2004;81(4):1151–3.

42. Gendall KA, Joyce PR, Carter FA, McIntosh VV, Bulik CM. Thyroid indices and treatment outcome in bulimia nervosa. Acta Psychiatr Scand. 2003;108(3):190–5.

43. Naessén S, Carlström C, Glant R, Jacobsson H, Hirschberg AL. Bone mineral density in bulimic women—influence of endocrine factors and previous anorexia. Eur J Endocrinol. 2006;155:245–51.

44. Hirschberg AL. Sex hormones, appetite and eating behaviour in women. Maturitas. 2012;71:248–56.

45. Azziz R, Carmina E, ZiJiang Chen Z, Dunaif A, Laven JSE, Legro RS, Lizneva D, Natterson-Horowtiz B, Teede HJ, Yildiz BO. Polycystic ovary syndrome. Nat Rev Dis Primers. 2016;2:16057.

46. Rotterdam ESHRE/ASRM-Sponsored PCOS Consensus Workshop Group. Revised 2003 consensus on diagnostic criteria and long-term health risks related to polycystic ovary syndrome. Fertil Steril. 2004;81:19–25.

47. Hirschberg AL, Naessén S, Stridsberg M, Byström B, Holte J. Impaired cholecystokinin secretion and disturbed appetite regulation in women with polycystic ovary syndrome. Gynecol Endocrinol. 2004;19:79–87.

48. Thannickal A, Brutocao C, Alsawas M, Morrow A, Zaiem F, Murad MH, Chattha AJ. Eating, sleeping and sexual function disorders in women with polycystic ovary syndrome (PCOS): a systematic review and meta-analysis. Clin Endocrinol (Oxf). 2020;92(4):338–49.
49. McCluskey SE, Lacey JH, Pearce JM. Binge-eating and polycystic ovaries. Lancet. 1992;340:723.
50. Morgan JF, McCluskey SE, Brunton JN, Hubert Lacey J. Polycystic ovarian morphology and bulimia nervosa: a 9-year follow-up study. Fertil Steril. 2002;77(5):928–31.
51. Naessén S, Garoff L, Carlström K, Glant R, Hirschberg AL. Polycystic ovary syndrome in bulimic women—an evaluation based on the new diagnostic criteria. Gynecol Endocrinol. 2006;22:388–94.
52. Eriksson E. Behavioral effects of androgens in women. In: Steiner M, Yonkers KA, Eriksson E, editors. Mood disorders in women. London: Martin Dunitz; 2000. p. 233–46.
53. Cooney LG, Dokras A. Depression and anxiety in polycystic ovary syndrome: etiology and treatment. Curr Psychiatry Rep. 2017;19(11):83.
54. Abraham S. Sexuality and reproduction in bulimia nervosa patients over 10 years. J Psychosom Res. 1998;44(3–4):491–502.
55. Johansen N, Hirschberg AL, Moen MH. The role of testosterone in menopausal hormone treatment. What is the evidence? Acta Obstet Gynecol Scand. 2020;99(8):966–9.
56. Sundblad C, Landén M, Eriksson T, Bergman L, Eriksson E. Effects of the androgen antagonist flutamide and the serotonin reuptake inhibitor citalopram in bulimia nervosa: a placebo-controlled pilot study. J Clin Psychopharmacol. 2005;25(1):85–8.
57. Naessén S, Carlström K, Byström B, Pierre Y, Hirschberg AL. Effects of an antiandrogenic oral contraceptive on appetite and eating behavior in bulimic women. Psychoneuroendocrinology. 2007;32(5):548–54.
58. Robinson L, Aldridge V, Clark EM, Misra M, Micali N. A systematic review and meta-analysis of the association between eating disorders and bone density. Osteoporos Int. 2016;27(6):1953–66.
59. Hagan KE, Walsh BT. State of the art: the therapeutic approaches to bulimia nervosa. Clin Ther. 2021;43(1):40–9.
60. Slade E, Keeney E, Mavranezouli I, Dias S, Fou L, Stockton S, Saxon L, Waller G, Turner H, Serpell L, Fairburn CG, Kendall T. Treatments for bulimia nervosa: a network meta-analysis. Psychol Med. 2018;48:2629–36.

The New Forms of Functional Hypothalamic Amenorrhoea

4

Vincenzina Bruni, Metella Dei, and Simona Ambroggio

4.1 Special Profiles of Functional Hypothalamic Amenorrhoea (FHA)

FHA is a heterogeneous form of primary or secondary amenorrhea, mainly related to behavioural factors, that involves reduction in hypothalamic gonadotropin-releasing hormone (GnRH) drive. The GnRH dysfunction impairs FSH and LH production and, consequently, ovarian function [1]. Low energy availability due to disorderly eating and excessive or nutritionally unbalanced physical activity together with stressful events or high vulnerability to psychosocial pressure are often interrelated causes of FHA.

A genetic susceptibility of the hypothalamic-pituitary-ovarian axis has also been demonstrated. Rare variants in genes associated with idiopathic hypogonadotropic hypogonadism, especially loss-of-function mutations of genes involved in GnRH ontogeny and function and its receptors, have been discovered [2]. Recently, these results have been confirmed and expanded through the use of more advanced genetic investigation techniques [3]. An increased genetic load of heterozygous rare sequence variants of genes encoding gonadotropic axis development and homeostasis increases the vulnerability to metabolic and psychological stressors that occur during or after puberty.

Adolescent and young people are more sensitive to negative consequences of stress exposure [4] and to endocrine repercussions of low energy availability [5].

V. Bruni (✉)
University of Florence, Florence, Italy

M. Dei
F.P. Florence, Florence, Italy

S. Ambroggio
F.P. Torino, Torino, Italy
e-mail: unknownddd@meteor.com

© International Society of Gynecological Endocrinology 2023   53
A. R. Genazzani et al. (eds.), *Amenorrhea*, ISGE Series,
https://doi.org/10.1007/978-3-031-22378-5_4

Thus, FHA is highly prevalent in the post-menarcheal years. Furthermore, prolonged oestrogen deficiency has a stronger impact on a growing organism. We underscore the repercussions on bone mass (especially the trabecular component) of low energy availability, hypercortisolaemia, and hypoestrogenemia during the critical time of skeletal accrual [6]. Several studies present evidences that link this condition to endothelial dysfunction and a premature increase of cardiovascular risk [7]. Chronic stress induces high systemic and cerebrospinal fluid levels of cortisol, toxic for neurons and glia in certain vulnerable areas of central nervous system. Low oestradiol concentrations potentiate the risk to brain health [8].

In the context of functional hypothalamic amenorrhoea, we will discuss three particular situations that sometimes may overlap:

(a) Borderline energy deficiency
(b) Persistent amenorrhoea after weight recovery
(c) FHA in subjects with polycystic ovary

We will start from a synthetic overview of endocrine mechanisms involved in the pathogenesis of menstrual dysfunction and adaptations to persistent reduction in energy availability and to chronic stressful situations, before facing the challenges of diagnostic evaluation of these specific clinical conditions.

4.2   The Crosstalk Between Body and Central Nervous System on Endocrine and Metabolic Homeostasis

The attainment and the maintenance of menstrual function, as a requisite of reproductive capacity, are gated by nutritional and metabolic cues [9], because the presence of sufficient energy reserves is critical to achieve successful reproduction. Several recent studies shed light on neuronal and endocrine components of the fine regulation of GnRH pulsatile secretion from hypothalamus, although a full understanding of all the actors involved in this mechanism is probably far to be attained.

The cell bodies of GnRH-secreting neurons are scattered in various hypothalamic nuclei; the majority reside in the arcuate (or infundibular) nucleus of the medial basal hypothalamus. Their axonal projections reach the median eminence, which abuts the hypothalamic-pituitary portal system. A complex neuronal network regulates the activity of GnRH neurons, through the interplay of stimulating and inhibiting factors (Fig. 4.1). Hypothalamic kisspeptin (KP) system is a key player in the central regulation of puberty and menstrual function. KP acts on specific KP receptors on GnRH nerve fibres, by intermittently stimulating their secretion and, consequently, pituitary LH release. In humans, hypothalamic KP neurons have been identified mainly in arcuate nucleus and preoptic region [10]; their axonal projection reaches the median eminence, an area exposed to blood circulation. In rodents and ruminants, this subpopulation of neurons co-expresses kisspeptin, neurokinin B, and dynorphin (abbreviated as KNDy neurons). Current data support the hypothesis that also in humans KNDy neurons represent the basic pulse-generating

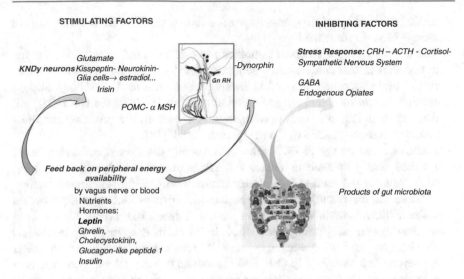

STIMULATING FACTORS

Glutamate
KNDy neurons Kisspeptin- Neurokinin-
Glia cells→ estradiol...
Irisin

POMC- α MSH

-Dynorphin

Gn RH

INHIBITING FACTORS

Stress Response: CRH – ACTH - Cortisol-
Sympathetic Nervous System

GABA
Endogenous Opiates

Feed back on peripheral energy availability
by vagus nerve or blood
Nutrients
Hormones:
Leptin
Ghrelin,
Cholecystokinin,
Glucagon-like peptide 1
Insulin

Products of gut microbiota

Fig. 4.1 Simplified outline of factors regulating gonadotropin-releasing hormone production and pulsatility

network in gonadotropin regulation, with a greater expression in women than in men. In animal models, the inhibiting effect of oestradiol and testosterone on KNDy neurons has been clearly demonstrated, supporting the notion that these neurons mediate the negative feedback action of gonadal steroids [11]. In regard to our topic, the most interesting studies are those focusing on the mechanisms underlying the metabolic regulation of KP system and other modulators of hypothalamic-pituitary-gonadal (HPG) axis. The role of KP system is to convey signals of metabolic homeostasis from the body to determine the appropriate pattern of GnRH release. This involves multiple mechanisms, still under investigation:

– The neuronal population in median eminence is directly exposed to circulating nutrients (glucose, few amino acids …) but also oleoylethanolamide and biliary acids produced by gut microbiota; this nutrient sensing enables the neurons to response in real time to metabolic changes, for instance modifying AMP kinase [12].
– The Kiss-1 gene expression may be regulated by epigenetic mechanisms, modifying the genome in response to behavioural or environmental factors, adapting transcriptional activity in response to metabolic signals [13]. Several gastrointestinal hormones (ghrelin, cholecystokinin, glucagon-like peptide 1 …) transmit signals involved in feeding and metabolic homeostasis to the brain via the vagal afferent system. KP neurons express receptors for various metabolic hormones: insulin, ghrelin, …, but their specific role in HPG activity maintenance is still speculative.
– Other neuromodulators involved in the control of food intake and energy expenditure (proopiomelanocortin, agouti-related protein) are probably involved, reg-

ulating the activity of KP neurons even if a direct action on KP neurons has not always been demonstrated.

- The status of energy reserve is another piece of essential information for the hypothalamus: this data is mainly communicated by leptin, an adipokine synthetized in fat tissue and secreted at levels proportional to the existing adipose storage. Leptin receptors are expressed at multiple levels of the HPG axis, KP neurons included, but ventral pre-mammillary neurons are probably the most involved in the mediation of leptin stimulus on KP [14].
- Irisin, encoded by the FNDC5 gene, is a recently discovered endocrine factor secreted mainly by skeletal muscle and adipose tissue, which increases during acute exercise and leads to energy expenditure by stimulating the transformation of white adipose tissue in brown adipose tissue. Irisin production and fat brown tissue activation modulate short-term glucose homeostasis, even if the involved mechanisms are not yet fully understood. In animal models, irisin expression has also been reported in hypothalamus where it exerts a stimulatory effect on GnRH expression and release [15]. One could speculate that central and peripheral irisin represents a link between body energy expenditure and hypothalamic control of feeding and menstrual function.
- Stress modulates GnRH secretion by activating the corticotrophin-releasing factor (CRF) system and sympatho-adrenal pathways, as well as the limbic brain. CRF is a potent inhibitor of the GnRH pulse generator, although the precise sites and mechanisms of action remain to be elucidated [16]. The negative effect on reproductive function is attributable in part to the increase in adrenally derived glucocorticoids, above all cortisol. In subjects with FHA, CSF cortisol concentrations were 30% greater when serum cortisol was 16% higher than in controls [17]. Cortisol has been reported to disrupt GnRH pulsatility and may have a direct action at the pituitary level.

4.3 Adaptation to Low Energy Availability (LEA) and to Persistent Psychological and Physical Stress

The adaptation of metabolic balance to nutrient intake is an essential ability for survival during caloric restriction or high-energy demand. During periods of prolonged LEA, it is mandatory to access energy storage tissues and reduce the overall body expenditure modulating thermogenesis, glucose utilization, and processes of tissue repair. All mitochondrial oxidative processes and consequently ATP production slow down. Thyroid hormones (TH) are the main regulators of energy expenditure. In situation of LEA, there is a reduction of de-iodination of thyroxine (T4) in 3-iodo-L-thyronine (T3), the more active hormone, in peripheral tissue. It has been experimentally calculated that this enzymatic modification occurs under the threshold of 25 kcal/kg lean body mass (LBM) per day [18] in subjects with elevated levels of physical activity than during caloric restriction. More recent findings indicate that TH actions on energy metabolism are mainly centrally mediated: T3 acts on the ventromedial nucleus of the hypothalamus to regulate thermogenesis in brown adipose tissue [19] and browning of white adipose tissue [20], by activating key lipogenic enzymes mediated by the sympathetic nervous system. Moreover, T3 regulates hepatic lipid oxidation through the vagus nerve. A central effect of TH has also been implicated in the regulation of glucose production and insulin sensitivity [21]. Low levels of T3 and its free form induce a generalized reduction of mitochondrial oxidative activity.

The negative energy balance in the liver reduces the production of insulin-like growth factor IGF-1, while growth hormone (GH) levels are increased, suggesting relative Gh resistance [22]. This is in general a marker of malnutrition. Gh also plays a direct metabolic role reducing insulin sensitivity and increasing lipolysis: neither of these effects are mediated by IGF-1 [23]. In individuals with LEA, Gh response to GhRH is increased; also, the levels of ghrelin (an orexigenic peptide secreted by stomach oxyntic cells, which physiologically stimulates Gh production) are raised. Gh pituitary release is also stimulated by intensive exercise.

The hepatic production of sex hormone-binding globulin decreases in situations of poor nutrient intake [24], parallel with the reduction of liver oxidative processes and of insulin release into the bloodstream. Low insulin levels are the result of both chronic undernutrition and heavy exercise.

A fall in circulating leptin occurs in a dose-response manner early during LEA status, well before there are measurable changes in fat mass. The interpretation of this finding is that leptin levels not only attempt to induce a state of positive energy balance but also activate an adaptive "starvation" response whose net effect is to conserve energy during times of privation [25]. Both dietary restriction and exercise have been related to decreases in circulating leptin, and the value of 30 Kcal/Kg LBM/day is always the threshold for this endocrine modification [26].

The exposure to stressful conditions induces the release of hypothalamic CRH, leading to increased pulses of adrenocorticotrophic hormone (ACTH) from the pituitary and glucocorticoid release from the adrenal glands and an activation of sympatho-adrenal medullary system with increased production of catecholamines. Although this acute hypothalamic-pituitary-adrenal (HPA) axis response to stressors is beneficial and helps the organism to cope with the situation, constant activation of this circuitry by chronic or traumatic stressful episodes may lead to a dysregulation of the axis and cause pathology. 24-h mean cortisol production and cortisol levels at night remain elevated during periods of prolonged psychological, physical, or metabolic stress, but the response to CRH administration becomes blunted. One systematic review demonstrated that caloric restriction per se significantly increases serum cortisol level, especially during fasting and in the initial period of dieting, but this modification tends to decrease after several weeks [27]. During undernutrition, cortisol also acts as a metabolic hormone stimulating hepatic gluconeogenesis to mobilize glucose and enhancing adipose tissue lipolysis. Highly trained athletes display decreased HPA response to exercise, but, on the other hand, exhibit a chronic mild hypercortisolism that may be an adaptive change to chronic physical activity in order to ensure homeostasis and promote anabolism [28].

In conclusion, endocrine-mediated metabolic adaptation to reduce total energy expenditure (EE) appears to be more specific to LEA related to caloric restriction, and it is minimally present in exercise-induced weight loss. However, hormonal repercussions of both strenuous physical activity and prolonged stress exposure tend to intensify the activity of the same endocrine and metabolic networks, with elevated inter-individual differences related to attitude to weight control and vulnerability to performance pressure.

4.4   Diagnostic Workup

FHA is a diagnosis of exclusion [1], and careful clinical history is valuable to guide this diagnostic evaluation. It is important to register the pubertal and menstrual history, but also to screen for current psychological stressors and for previous events, with particular attention to conditioning high stress sensitivity. The use of a validated questionnaire, as the Perceived Stress Scale [29], may help. Specific attitudes such as perfectionism, expectations for herself and others, and a high need for social approval should also be investigated. A part of the history should focus on diet, food selectivity and ideologies, previous eating disorders, weight changes, as well as exercise (type, duration, and intensity) or athletic training. Other questions should inquire about the presence of headache, bowel habits, and use of laxatives, diuretics, or dietary supplements.

A full physical examination, including the measurement of body mass index (BMI), blood pressure, and heart rate, and a gynaecological examination, is necessary. A US pelvic scan may add further information on the functional status of uterus and ovaries [30]. In particular, the measurement of endometrial thickness is an indirect evaluation of oestrogen levels and may substitute for MPA test: 6 mm of endometrial lining corresponds with bleeding after 10 mg of dydrogesterone for 5 days [31]. The presence and dimensions of follicles inside the ovaries represent a less univocal marker of residual function.

Initial blood workup should include measurement of the beta subunit of human chorionic gonadotropin concentration, regardless of the sexual history, to rule out pregnancy. Early-morning FSH, LH, prolactin, oestradiol, AMH, TSH, and T4 should be measured routinely. If history suggests a deficiency in energy availability, it is useful to check metabolic hormones: FT3, IGF-1, insulin together with glucose levels, and, if possible, leptin. Assessment of cortisol status may also be considered, keeping in mind that salivary cortisol is a better biomarker than serum cortisol; in any case, so many factors are involved in modulating HPA axis reactivity that a linear relationship between CRH-ACTH production and cortisol in blood or urine or other body compartments does not necessarily exist [32]. The dosage of total immunoglobulin A and of anti-transglutaminase antibodies rules out coeliac disease.

General laboratory tests with complete blood count, chemistry and liver panel, and C-reactive protein are seldom in the normal range. We have to consider with attention:

- Plasma proteins because albumin tends to decrease during fasting
- Ferritin because levels are high in inflammatory states
- Retinol-binding protein, pre-albumin, and transferrin determinations that are sensitive indicators only in severe protein malnutrition

- Leukopenia, sometimes related to LEA
- Hypercholesterolaemia as a marker of mobilization of fat stores
- Increased liver enzymes, especially aspartate aminotransferase (AST), as a result of hepatic impairment related to energy deficiency
- Hypokalaemia mainly related to bulimic behaviours

Bone mineral density (BMD) measurement by dual-energy X-ray absorptiometry (DXA) is required for any adolescent or woman with 6 or more months of amenorrhoea. With total body DXA, an evaluation of body composition is possible with the assessment of fat mass and lean body mass for the total body and single districts. A simplified measure of body composition can be obtained using body impedance analysis (BIA), a test that consents easy repetitions of the measurements over time. Lean body mass is the most relevant tissue pool for energy availability, which increases in the first gynaecological years in all subjects [33], but it becomes particularly prevalent in athletes. Body fat reference curves teach us that whole-body fat percentage in girls after menarche displays a very wide inter-individual variability, ranging for instance in years from 21 to 28 in 16-year-olds [34].

4.5 Special Clinical Situations in the Framework of FHA

The sociocultural pressure to be thin very often induces in adolescent and young adult females to experience body dissatisfaction and a habit of various weight control behaviours: occasional fasting, "yo-yo" dieting, and use of drugs reducing fat absorption. The same thin-ideal image often leads to exercising for physical fitness, which may become an addiction, enhanced by the use of fitness trackers. Thus, many young women, even if they do not fulfil the psychopathological profile of well-defined eating disorders, spend years of their life struggling for a presumed "healthy" lifestyle that is ultimately an intermittent control on body energy homeostasis. The menstrual function, especially in individuals more sensitive to the impact of metabolic or psychological stress on hypothalamic regulation, reacts with periods of oligo-menorrhoea or secondary amenorrhoea.

The problem is how to identify these clinical situations related to chronic mildly reduced energy availability or to intermittent LEA. A thorough interview regarding individual behaviour and underlying motivations usually sets off the first alarm. BMI is often normal and, especially in exercising subjects, is not a valid marker of hypo-metabolic state [35]. Considering the endocrine profile, gonadotropin levels are often normal and even the metabolic hormones (FT3, IGF-1, insulin) may result near to the lower limit of the normal range but may not be clearly diagnostic. There is little data on the sensitivity of serum leptin in the identification of subclinical LEA; the dosage of kisspeptin is under study [36]. An evaluation of body composition may help [37]: we can use BIA to measure fat-free mass and fat mass, bearing in mind the fact that the estimate of fat stores is indirect, as a difference between weight and fat-free mass. BIA underestimates fat mass in comparison with the direct measure of DXA, while overestimates lean mass, because the measure

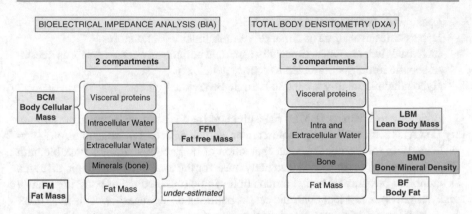

Fig. 4.2 Measurement of body composition: comparison between BIA and total body DXA

includes bone (Fig. 4.2). The FM cut-off for menstrual function is not defined; we estimate values around 17–18%. Regarding lean mass, BIA evidences body mass cells (BMC), the more active metabolic component, which is primarily affected in hypo-metabolic states. Body cell mass indexed to height (BCMI) is a good proxy of the state of nutrition, and an index <7 is considered a clear marker of malnutrition, but a reading of this value as a continuous variable may prove useful. Another interesting datum is phase angle, a marker of water distribution between intra- and extracellular spaces, that tends to reduce in situations of LEA, and it is a predictor of resting energy expenditure (REE) [38]. DXA is the technique of reference for the assessment of body composition in clinical practice. The healthy cut-off of percentage fat mass is not univocal, but we estimate 18–19% as a possible threshold. Indirect evidence derives from the study on constitutional thinness, defined as a state of severe underweight with a body mass index similar to anorectic patients in the absence of any eating disorders or other obvious disruptive factors affecting energy balance. These subjects present fat mass over 18% while fat-free mass is reduced [39]. Moreover, concerning the attainment of menarche, differences between upper- and lower-body (gluteal-femoral) fat seem significant, suggesting that fat distribution may be more relevant than total fat [40]. It may be advisable to study district fat accumulation also in women of reproductive age.

Another approach to the identification of borderline situations of energy deficiency is the measurement of resting energy expenditure (REE), that is, the amount of calories required for a 24-h period by the body during a non-active period. It is a component of total daily EE (Fig. 4.3) plus diet-induced thermogenesis and physical activity-related EE, which is proportional to body mass and is reduced in metabolic adaptation to low-energy states. REE is measured by indirect calorimetry either with a bedside ventilated hood system or in a whole-room metabolic chamber [41]; it can be estimated by numerous formulas, taking into account weight, height, and age or derived by body composition measurements. This index is widely used in sport medicine [42], but it should be used also in other subjects with menstrual disturbances.

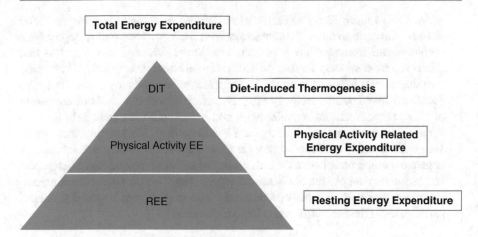

Fig. 4.3 Components of total daily energy expenditure

If a study of body composition and metabolic adaptation to energy restriction is probably the key for highlighting subclinical LEA, consideration of these factors may also be useful in the clinical setting of persistent amenorrhoea in eating disorders after weight recovery. Researchers have proposed various factors as predictive of menstrual recovery after weight gain [43]:

- BMI, based on the population standard for age, is an inadequate marker. The BMI value before the onset of amenorrhoea is more significant [44].
- Stored body fat could be another important step. A meta-analysis of seven selected studies [45] comprising 366 adolescent and young adult females with anorexia nervosa revealed that patients who resumed their menstrual cycle had a significantly higher mean % BF when compared to those who did not (SMD: 3.74, 95% CI: 2.26–5.22). % BF was found to be an independent predictor of the recovery of menses, and an increase of a single unit of % BF can increase the odds of menstruation by ≈15–20%. The authors suggested a cut-off point of % BF ≈21 as the minimum needed for menstrual function. It is important to do the assessment in a clinical setting, especially after complete weight restoration. A similar threshold (21% of fat mass) has been identified, using BIA, as the most discriminant for menstrual resumption compared with other anthropometric parameters in adolescents who have recovered from anorexia nervosa [46].
- Resting energy expenditure, as a measure of hypo-metabolic state, is lower in weight-restored subjects with amenorrhoea than in subjects who are menstruating normally [47].
- The normalization of metabolic hormones (FT3, insulin, IGF-1, and leptin) is a prerequisite for the recovery of pulsatile function of GnRH, but it is not always predictive of restoration of menstrual function.
- Psycho-relational well-being is a complex variable associated with the outcome of restrictive eating disorders. In a cohort study of Finnish twins [48], unrecovered

women were more likely to suffer from depressive symptoms prior to eating disorder onset, to express dissatisfaction with their partners, and to report high perfectionism than recovered women. One systematic review evidenced that minimal persistent food control, difficulties in self-acceptance, and building new meaningful relationships were the current factors significantly associated with decreased likelihood of recovery [49]. Direct endocrine diagnosis of activation of stress response is not reliable, but a competent interview may help to draw attention to these aspects. A study on 71 patients with FHA demonstrated that kisspeptin and LH continue to rely on kisspeptin to drive GnRH discharge. A negative correlation between the concentration and pulse frequency of kisspeptin and serum cortisol plasma levels has been observed. This is another elegant demonstration that HPA axis activation, in response to persistent stressful situation, participates in the functional reproductive blockade [50].

Choice of appropriate intervention, including eventual prescription of transdermal E2 therapy associated with cyclic oral progestin, to help young women who continue to have amenorrhoea even after nutritional rehabilitation, modified exercise intensity, and psychotherapy depends on the evaluation of all the above variables. We note that randomized controlled trials have reported positive effects of physiologic oestrogen replacement on bone loss that is probably the more dangerous long-term effect of FHA [51].

Another clinical possibility with clear impact on the recovery of menstrual function is the possible coexistence of polycystic ovary syndrome or hyperinsulinaemia and restrictive eating disorders. These subjects may be identified during diagnostic workup from clinical history: young women with signs of androgen excess and/or glucose dysmetabolism who started on a hypocaloric diet and a programme of physical activity as a treatment. We know well that if external stressors and personal concern about body image are present, it is very easy to drift to pathological weight control behaviours.

A few studies have shown that these women may have some endocrine features of polycystic ovary syndrome, together with those of FHA. These features include an increased androgen response to gonadotropins and sometimes androgen levels in the upper normal range or slightly elevated despite low or normal gonadotropin and increased anti-Mullerian hormone levels [52]. Ovarian volume is increased, and a polycystic ovarian morphology (PCOM) is often present. We would stress that a multifollicular ovarian morphology without increased stromal echogenicity is quite frequent in FHA and probably represents a marker of immaturity or of functional regression [53], which can be associated with slightly elevated AMH levels. This ultrasonographic finding may be confused with a typical polycystic ovary, where the increased number of small follicles is associated with evidence of the stromal component and consequently enlarged dimensions. Thus, the suspicion of underlying polycystic ovary syndrome should not be based on this variable alone. After weight recovery, LH value often remains in the upper range.

Persisting hypo-metabolic state in subjects with poor metabolic flexibility, related to insulin resistance, probably explains the difficulties in reaching a condition of physiological homeostasis with nutritional rehabilitation. Various studies have demonstrated that in all women with restrictive eating disorders, refeeding is associated with an increase in abdominal fat, which might be responsible for a reduction in insulin sensitivity [54]. The increase in visceral adiposity is associated with an abnormal glucose response during OGTT even in women who do not develop overt insulin resistance [55]. A personal genetic or epigenetic trend to glucose dysmetabolism may exacerbate this transient step of recovery. Therefore, competent counselling on current eating habits and lifestyle changes and an estimate of visceral fat are mandatory in dealing with these subjects. Further clinical studies on this specific condition are necessary to prepare an outline of specific items of attention for therapeutic projects regarding this subgroup of patients. In a small follow-up study, the features related to the tendency to PCOS appear to be reversible after menstrual recovery [56].

In conclusion, FHA is a wide definition, including menstrual dysfunction related to different causes and with a variable impact of psychological stress, food attitudes, and energy drainage due to physical activity. Identification of the burden of various components and their evolution over time is important both for explaining the situation to the patient and tailoring therapeutic strategies which are often multi-professional.

References

1. Gordon CM, Ackerman KE, Berga SL, Kaplan JR, et al. Functional hypothalamic amenorrhea: an Endocrine Society clinical practice guideline. J Clin Endocrinol Metab. 2017;102:1413–9.
2. Caronia LM, Martin C, Welt CK, et al. A genetic basis for functional hypothalamic amenorrhea. N Engl J Med. 2011;364(3):215–25.
3. Delaney A, Burkholder AB, Lavender CA, et al. Increased burden of rare sequence variants in GnRH associated genes in women with hypothalamic amenorrhea. J Clin Endocrinol Metab. 2020;106(3):e1441–552.
4. Romeo RD. Adolescence: a central event in shaping stress reactivity. Dev Psychobiol. 2010;52(3):244–53.
5. Loucks AB. The response of luteinizing hormone pulsatility to 5 days of low energy availability disappears by 14 years of gynecological age. J Clin Endocrinol Metab. 2006;91(8):3158–64.
6. Mitchell DM, Tuck P, Ackerman KE, et al. Altered trabecular bone morphology in adolescent and young adult athletes with menstrual dysfunction. Bone. 2015;81:24–30.
7. Shufelt C, Torbati T, Dutra E. Hypothalamic amenorrhea and the long-term consequences. Semin Reprod Med. 2017;35(3):256–62.
8. Prokai D, Berga SL. Neuroprotection via reduction in stress: altered menstrual patterns as a marker for stress and implications for long-term neurologic health in women. Int J Mol Sci. 2016;17:2147–53.
9. Tena-Sempere M. Neuroendocrinology in 2016: neuroendocrine control of metabolism and reproduction. Nat Rev Endocrinol. 2017;13(2):67–8.
10. Hrabovsky R. Neuroanatomy of human kisspeptin system. Neuroendocrinology. 2014;99:33–48.
11. Lehman MN, He W, Coolen LM, et al. Does the KNDy model for the control of gonadotropin-releasing hormone pulses apply to monkeys and humans? Semin Reprod Med. 2019;37:71–83.
12. Hardie DG, Ross FA, Hawley SA. AMPK: a nutrient and energy sensor that maintains energy v homeostasis. Nat Rev Mol Cell Biol. 2012;13:251–62.

13. Navarro VM. Metabolic regulation of kisspeptin—the link between energy balance and reproduction. Nat Rev Endocrinol. 2020;16(8):407–20.
14. Childs GV, Odle AK, MacNicol MC, et al. The importance of leptin to reproduction. Endocrinology. 2021;162(2):bqaa204.
15. Wahab F, Khan IU, Polo IR, Zubair H, et al. Irisin in the primate hypothalamus and its effect on GnRH in vitro. J Endocrinol. 2019;241(3):175–87.
16. Li XF, Knox AM, O'Byrne KT. Corticotrophin-releasing factor and stress-induced inhibition of the gonadotrophin-releasing hormone pulse generator in the female. Brain Res. 2010;1364:153–63.
17. Brundu B, Loucks TL, Adler LJ, et al. Increased cortisol in the cerebrospinal fluid of women with functional hypothalamic amenorrhea. J Clin Endocrinol Metab. 2006;91(4):1561–5.
18. Loucks AB, Heath EM. Induction of low-T3 syndrome in exercising women occurs at a threshold of energy availability. Am J Physiol. 1994;266(3 Pt 2):R817–23.
19. López M, Varela L, Vázquez MJ, et al. Hypothalamic AMPK and fatty acid metabolism mediate thyroid regulation of energy balance. Nat Med. 2010;16(9):1001–8.
20. Martínez-Sánchez N, Moreno-Navarrete JM, Contreras C, et al. Thyroid hormones induce browning of white fat. J Endocrinol. 2017;232(2):351–62.
21. Zhang Z, Boelen A, Bisschop PH, et al. Hypothalamic effects of thyroid hormone. Mol Cell Endocrinol. 2017;15(458):143–8.
22. Fleming S, Morrison AE, Levy MJ. A review of the pathophysiology of functional hypothalamic amenorrhoea in women subject to psychological stress, disordered eating, excessive exercise or a combination of these factors. Clin Endocrinol (Oxf). 2021;95(2):229–38.
23. Mauras N, Haymond MW. Are the metabolic effects of GH and IGF-I separable? Growth Horm IGF Res. 2005;15(1):19–27.
24. Barbe P, Bennet A, Stebenet M, et al. Sex-hormone-binding globulin and protein-energy malnutrition indexes as indicators of nutritional status in women with anorexia nervosa. Am J Clin Nutr. 1993;57(3):319–22.
25. Friedman JM. Leptin and the endocrine control of energy balance. Nat Metab. 2019;1(8):754–64.
26. Hilton LK, Loucks AB. Low energy availability, not exercise stress, suppresses the diurnal rhythm of leptin in healthy young women. Am J Physiol Endocrinol Metab. 2000;278:E43–9.
27. Nakamura Y, Walker BR, Ikuta T. Systematic review and meta-analysis reveals acutely elevated plasma cortisol following fasting but not less severe calorie restriction. Stress. 2016;19(2):151–7.
28. Mastorakos G, Pavlatou M, Diamanti-Kandarakis E, et al. Exercise and the stress system. Hormones. 2005;4(2):73–89.
29. Cohen S, Williamson G. Perceived stress in a probability sample of the United States. In: Spacapan S, Oskamp S, editors. The social psychology of health. Newbury Park: Sage; 1988.
30. Teo SI, Chong CL. A systematic approach to imaging the pelvis in amenorrhea. Abdom Radiol (NY). 2021;46(7):3326–41.
31. Nakamura S, Douchi T, Oki T, et al. Relationship between sonographic endometrial thickness and progestin-induced withdrawal bleeding. Obstet Gynecol. 1996;87(5 Pt 1):722–5.
32. Hellhammer DH, Wüst S, Kudielka BM. Salivary cortisol as a biomarker in stress research. Psychoneuroendocrinology. 2009;34(2):163–71.
33. Bandini LG, Must A, Naumova EN, et al. Change in leptin, body composition and other hormones around menarche—a visual representation. Acta Paediatr. 2008;97:1454–9.
34. McCarthy HD, Cole TJ, Fry T, et al. Body fat reference curves for children. Int J Obes. 2006;30:598–602.
35. Klungland Torstveit M, Sundgot-Borgen J. Are under- and overweight female elite athletes thin and fat? A controlled study. Med Sci Sports Exerc. 2012;44(5):949–57.
36. Bacopoulou F, Lambrou GI, Rodanaki ME, et al. Serum kisspeptin concentrations are negatively correlated with body mass index in adolescents with anorexia nervosa and amenorrhea. Hormones (Athens). 2017;16(1):33–41.
37. Bruni V, Dei M, Morelli C, et al. Body composition variables and leptin levels in functional hypothalamic amenorrhea and amenorrhea related to eating disorders. J Pediatr Adolesc Gynecol. 2011;24(6):347–52.

38. Marra M, Di Vincenzo V, Cioffi I, et al. Resting energy expenditure in elite athletes: development of new predictive equations based on anthropometric variables and bioelectrical impedance analysis derived phase angle. J Int Soc Sports Nutr. 2021;18(1):68.
39. Bailly M, Boscaro A, Pereira B, et al. Underweight but not underfat: is fat-free mass a key factor in constitutionally thin women? Eur J Clin Nutr. 2021;75(12):1764–70.
40. Lassek WD, Gaulin SJC. Brief communication: menarche is related to fat distribution. Am J Phys Anthropol. 2007;133(4):1147–51.
41. Lam YY, Ravussin E. Analysis of energy metabolism in humans: a review of methodologies. Mol Metab. 2016;5(11):1057–71.
42. Strock NCA, Koltun KJ, Southmayd EA, et al. Indices of resting metabolic rate accurately reflect energy deficiency in exercising women. Int J Sport Nutr Exerc Metab. 2020;30(1):14–24.
43. Pape J, Herbison AE, Leeners B. Recovery of menses after functional hypothalamic amenorrhoea: if, when and why. Hum Reprod Update. 2021;27(1):130–53.
44. Dei M, Seravalli V, Bruni V, et al. Predictors of recovery of ovarian function after weight gain in subjects with amenorrhea related to restrictive eating disorders. Gynecol Endocrinol. 2008;24(8):459–64.
45. Traboulsi S, Itani L, Tannir H, et al. Is body fat percentage a good predictor of menstrual recovery in females with anorexia nervosa after weight restoration? A systematic review and exploratory and selective meta-analysis. J Popul Ther Clin Pharmacol. 2019;26(2):e25–37.
46. Tokatly Latzer I, Kidron-Levy H, Stein D, et al. Predicting menstrual recovery in adolescents with anorexia nervosa using body fat percent estimated by bioimpedance analysis. J Adolesc Health. 2019;64(4):454–60.
47. Sterling WM, Golden NH, Jacobson MS, et al. Metabolic assessment of menstruating and non-menstruating normal weight adolescents. Int J Eat Disord. 2009;42(7):658–63.
48. Keski-Rahkonen A, Raevuori A, Bulik CM, et al. Factors associated with recovery from anorexia nervosa: a population-based study. Int J Eat Disord. 2014;47(2):117–23.
49. Stockford C, Stenfert Kroese B, Beesley A, et al. Women's recovery from anorexia nervosa: a systematic review and meta-synthesis of qualitative research. Eat Disord. 2019;27(4):343–36.
50. Podfigurna A, Maciejewska-Jeske M, Meczekalski B, et al. Kisspeptin and LH pulsatility in patients with functional hypothalamic amenorrhea. Endocrine. 2020;70:635–43.
51. Robinson L, Micali N, Misra M. Eating disorders and bone metabolism in women. Curr Opin Pediatr. 2017;29(4):488–96.
52. Carmina E, Fruzzetti F, Lobo RA. Increased anti-Mullerian hormone levels and ovarian size in a subgroup of women with functional hypothalamic amenorrhea: further identification of the link between polycystic ovary syndrome and functional hypothalamic amenorrhea. Am J Obstet Gynecol. 2016;214(6):714.e1–6.
53. Villa P, Rossodivita A, Fulghesu AM. Insulin and GH secretion in adolescent girls with irregular cycles: polycystic vs multifollicular ovaries. J Endocrinol Invest. 2003;26(4):305–11.
54. Prioletta A, Muscogiuri G, Sorice GP, et al. In anorexia nervosa, even a small increase in abdominal fat is responsible for the appearance of insulin resistance. Clin Endocrinol (Oxf). 2011;75(2):202–6.
55. Kim Y, Hildebrandt T, Mayer LES. Differential glucose metabolism in weight restored women with anorexia nervosa. Psychoneuroendocrinology. 2019;110:104404.
56. Carmina E, Fruzzetti F, Lobo RA. Features of polycystic ovary syndrome (PCOS) in women with functional hypothalamic amenorrhea (FHA) may be reversible with recovery of menstrual function. Gynecol Endocrinol. 2018;34(4):301–4.

Exercise and Stress-Related Amenorrhea

5

Alessandro D. Genazzani, Tabatha Petrillo,
Nicola Piacquadio, Alessandra Sponzilli, Veronica Tomatis,
Fedora Ambrosetti, Melania Arnesano, Elisa Semprini,
Christian Battipaglia, and Tommaso Simoncini

5.1 Introduction

In these last decades, physical activity has been growing in interest both in men and in women as demonstrated by the increased number of participants to almost all casual and competitive sports such as the half-marathons or the marathons. Recent papers reported that in the USA among the finishers of the marathons, 40% of them were women [1]. Such reports clearly give an insight on the fact that more women than men have started to be physically active. It is out of any doubt that physical exercise gives and offers a lot of benefits in terms of health, but on the other hand excessive physical activity can induce adverse effects on some physical issues and on fertility. In fact, a higher incidence of reproductive problems has been reported to occur in athletes than in nonathletes, though training [2, 3] and more hours of intense physical activity have been associated with a reduced ovulating ability [4]. These facts clearly support the concept that increased frequency and duration/intensity of physical activity determine a greater difficulty in conceiving around 3.2-fold greater than the normal population [1, 5].

The reproductive impairments are not the only one that might be induced by excessive training. In fact, the female athlete triad (triad) is the classic clinical situation that most of these women might suffer. It usually hits women participating or training in high-intensity sports, and it is characterized by the presence of interrelated conditions: disordered eating, amenorrhea, and osteoporosis [6, 7]. Few years

A. D. Genazzani (✉) · T. Petrillo · N. Piacquadio · A. Sponzilli · V. Tomatis
F. Ambrosetti · M. Arnesano · E. Semprini · C. Battipaglia
Gynecological Endocrinology Center, Department of Obstetrics and Gynecology,
University of Modena and Reggio Emilia, Modena, Italy
e-mail: algen@unimo.it; fedora.ambrosetti01@universitadipavia.it

T. Simoncini
Department of Obstetrics and Gynecology, University of Pisa, Pisa, Italy
e-mail: tommaso.simoncini@med.unipi.it

© International Society of Gynecological Endocrinology 2023
A. R. Genazzani et al. (eds.), *Amenorrhea*, ISGE Series,
https://doi.org/10.1007/978-3-031-22378-5_5

ago, this definition was updated so that to involve any one of the three components: low energy availability (with/without eating disorder), menstrual dysfunction, and low bone mineral density (BMD) [8].

It comes clear from this that sport activity is able, when exaggerated, to affect not only the reproductive health but also the skeleton and bone metabolism. Christo et al. [9] reported that amenorrheic adolescent endurance runners had lower BMD than eumenorrheic runners and nonathletes. In addition, athletes have an additional clinical sign, that is, anemia, which occurs at a very high grade with hemoglobin levels <11.6 g/dL and iron deficiency [10] that are both direct and indirect effectors of the reduced athletic performances.

It comes clear that excessive training, improved energy expenditure, and altered feeding are at the basis of a non-well-structured biological health and from this fact comes out a reduced reproductive ability.

5.2   Menstrual Dysfunctions in Athletes

The real problem for women that exercise a lot is the menstrual regularity and the amount of bleeding. At our outpatient ambulatory, these kind of patients refer usually that the menstrual bleeding changed across the time and from regular it became less frequent and/or scarce and later amenorrhea occurred. In fact, the amenorrheic condition is the final end of such reproductive impairment that occurs in up to 44% of the athletes especially in those that need a light weight to better perform, such as dancers or short-distance runners [1, 11].

Though there is not a so vast literature, reports clearly indicate that such menstrual abnormality is mainly due to a luteal phase defect [12] greatly induced by the concomitant effects of psychological stress and metabolic stress, the latter due to the perfect combination of reduced amount of food and of specific nutrients (very often proteins) and excess energy consumption with training.

It is quite obvious the reason for which the luteal phase becomes insufficient or defective: abnormal neuroendocrine regulation of the GnRH release from hypothalamic neurons due to specific negative neuroendocrine and metabolic signals reduces the biological ability of GnRH to adequately stimulate the gonadotrope cells. Such a condition occurs with a relative rapidity, few weeks or months, determining the lack of gonadotropin stimulation on granulosa cells at the ovarian level. Recruitment and/or maturation of the ovarian follicles become slower or do not occur efficiently, thus determining an inadequate follicular phase and follicular growth with a subsequent anovulation. Such a picture determines a low growth of estradiol plasma levels with a subsequent inadequate progesterone secretion. In other words, the follicular phase becomes longer for the not efficient follicle growth and the luteal phase shortens, 10 days or less, and shows low or very low progesterone plasma levels since the ovarian cycle has been anovulatory [13]. A lot of runners and athletes suffer from this abnormal ovarian cycle despite showing menstrual bleeding. After some time, with persisting stressors, the ovarian cycle definitively fails to start due to the hypothalamic blockade of the GnRH release [14–16].

5.3 Training, Stress, and Altered Neuroendocrine Control of Reproduction

The physical, psychological, and metabolic conditions that negatively act centrally at the hypothalamic level on GnRH-secreting neuron level are identified as "stressors." One of the key events of this modulatory action is played by neurotransmitters and neuropeptides produced in the central nervous system. These neuronal pathways are sensitive to external and internal environmental changes (light-dark cycle, temperature) as well as to cognitive, social, cultural, and emotional events. Each of these signals may become stressor agents when acute changes occur, and through the integration with hormonal signals, they can stimulate adaptive responses.

Such negative hypothalamic response to stressors is nothing else than a defensive system. In human females, the adaptive mechanism during stress is represented by the reduction of reproductive axis activity, blocking a function which is considered not relevant to survive. Usually, poly- or oligomenorrhea may occur as an intermediate step that anticipates the amenorrheic condition, which is the final end of this clinical adaptive response to stress.

This adaptive response is not so mysterious and represents a normal response, with our biology being not so much different from the one that the human species had 20,000–30,000 years ago. In fact, though evolution permitted our species to change and to evolve as primates and bipeds, our neuroendocrine systems apparently still work and act similarly to a primate [17].

This means that whatever stressor of the twenty-first century (dieting, sport, training, or psychological stressors) hits the human being, the adaptive response is similar to the one that might be induced by the sight or the attack of a wild animal or by lack of food or by strenuous fatigue due to a migration [17].

5.4 Neuroendocrine Mechanisms of Stress-Induced Impairment of Reproductive Function

In experimental animals as well as in humans, the response to stressors is represented by the increase of adrenocorticotropic hormone (ACTH) and cortisol plasma levels. Since corticotropin-releasing hormone (corticotropin-releasing factor (CRF)) is the specific hypothalamic stimulating factor for ACTH, elevation of ACTH in response to stress is anticipated by the elevation of CRF stimulation. In fact, the intraventricular injection of CRF blunts GnRH and LH release [18, 19]. The use of CRF antagonists reverses the stress-induced LH decrease in rats [18]. The elevation of CRF as an adaptive response to stress occurs together with the increase of central ß-endorphin (ßEP) release, which is released when pro-opiomelanocortin (POMC) peptide is cleaved to release ACTH. ßEP is the most important peptide of the endogenous opioid peptide (EOP) family and is a potent inhibitor of GnRH-LH secretion. On such basis, the linkage between the activation of the hypothalamic-pituitary-adrenal (HPA) axis and the stress-induced inhibitory effects on the hypothalamic-pituitary-gonadal (HPG) axis is now clear [20]. Since naloxone, a specific opioid receptor antagonist, is able to counteract the CRF-induced LH secretory blockade [21], opioid peptides have been considered the key factor of the stress-induced inhibition of the HPG axis.

Other than adrenal gland hormones (i.e., cortisol), also prolactin (PRL) is activated by stress and both are able to act as stress-induced hormonal signal. In fact, cortisol negatively acts at the pituitary level on GnRH-stimulated LH release in rats [22]. PRL increases after stressful stimuli, such as emotional and physical events as well as internal rhythms such as sleep, and depends on the activation of several stimulating factors like thyrotropin-releasing hormone, vasoactive intestinal peptide, and oxytocin or failure of the dopaminergic control. Also, PRL negatively acts on the neuroendocrine modulation of GnRH-secreting neurons [17] and with the increased cortisol secretion participates in the negative effect both on gonadotropin secretion and on gonadal steroid biosynthesis. It has to be pointed out that when dealing with stressful situations affecting the reproductive axis, the real relevant ones are those that are chronically occurring, taking place several times all along the days and/or the weeks so that to become a constant negative trigger of the stress-induced endocrine response. Acute and rare or sporadic stressors (once in a week or so), despite altering the stress-induced hormone secretions, are not enough repetitive and/or strong to induce changes on the reproductive function.

An additional observation has to be done about the meaning of the elevation of cortisol in the patients hit by persistent stressful situations. The role of cortisol is quite important in the biology of primates, and it has a relevant role in humans. Stress-induced cortisol secretion is not merely related to the inhibition of GnRH secretion but also to the activation of gluconeogenesis, which represents the endogenous production of glucose from fat acids and from proteins. This event has a relevant biological meaning since it determines the production of glucose and energy degrading fat acids and proteins avoiding to claim for energy from fat (it would take lot of time), especially if being in dangerous situations. During stress, the increase of cortisol and PRL plasma levels is just below the higher levels of normality [16], but when insulin and fT3 plasma levels fall below the level of normality, the latter endocrine sign strongly supports the presence of chronic stressors and a metabolic impairment with reduced/abnormal feeding and/or excessive energy consumption. All these are endocrine markers of the activation due to stress of a complex compensatory and defensive system.

5.5   Neuroendocrine Mechanism of Hypothalamic Amenorrhea

Functional hypothalamic amenorrhea (FHA) [23–27] is the classic clinical situation that occurs in athletes or dancers consuming a lot of energy and not having an adequate caloric and nutritional intake. FHA is a model of hypoestrogenic condition characterized by several neuroendocrine aberrations which occur after a relatively long period of time of exposure to a repetitive and/or chronic stressor(s) so that to affect the neuroendocrine hypothalamic activity [26, 27] and the release of several hypophyseal hormones [14, 20] and among them those driving the reproductive axis.

In patients with FHA, the amenorrheic conditions are absolutely not related to organic diseases affecting the hypothalamus or the pituitary or the ovary. It comes out that the true FHA is diagnosed with a diagnosis of exclusion, through a well-structured anamnestic analysis considering the lifestyle also.

Being patients with FHA greatly under stress, as demonstrated in experimental animals, the EOPs exert an inhibitory effect on the episodic release of both GnRH and LH [28–30]. It is of interest to know that FHA is not responsive to naloxone infusion [31, 32], but after 2 months of hormonal replacement therapy, LH response to naloxone was recovered in at least 53% of the patients [33]. This fact sustains the hypothesis that a tight relationship links opioidergic system with gonadal steroids, especially estrogens [34]. In fact, when performing the naloxone infusion, it induces LH plasma level increase during the late follicular and luteal phases of the menstrual cycle but not during the early follicular phase [30, 35]. Such evidences clearly suggest that a specific estrogenic milieu is needed to have a specific modulation of the opioid receptor antagonist on opioidergic receptors. In fact, during postmenopause, the naloxone administration does not induce any LH release, but such response shows up when patients undergo estradiol administration, thus having a reduction of LH plasma levels and restoration of naloxone-induced LH response [34].

Other than the opioidergic system, also the dopaminergic and serotoninergic are involved in the negative modulation of GnRH release in FHA. When dopamine receptors are blocked by metoclopramide administration, the LH plasma levels increase in women with FHA but not in healthy eumenorrheic subjects [36], thus supporting the evidence of an impaired dopaminergic activity in stress-induced amenorrhea. Fenfluramine administration, a serotoninergic agonist, blunts cortisol response in FHA [37, 38], thus supporting the hypothesis that serotonin participates in the stress-induced neuroendocrine events leading to the HPA axis impaired activity. Probably, FHA patients have a reduced serotoninergic tone that interacts with EOPs in the regulation of the spontaneous GnRH-induced LH release. This interaction between the opioidergic and serotoninergic axes is supported by the fact that in normal subjects fenfluramine administration blocks the naloxone-induced LH secretion and determines the significant increase of plasma ACTH and cortisol plasma levels [37, 38]. However, even though the administration of cyproheptadine clorhydrate, a serotonin receptor antagonist, at the dose of 4 mg/day has been demonstrated to be effective in increasing LH, FSH, GH, and fT3 plasma levels, no effect of cyproheptadine was observed in naloxone-induced LH response in patients with HA [39].

5.6   Metabolic Signals as Stressors in Hypothalamic Amenorrhea

The mechanisms by which undernutrition and/or energy consumption act and determine the blockade of the central drive of the reproductive axis are complex and probably also involve not yet known pathways. However, a link exists between the reproductive dysfunctions and the severity of body weight loss [40, 41]. A key factor for the induction of the blockade of the reproductive axis is the percentage of body fat lost. Well-established data clearly suggest that the suppression of the neuroendocrine drive of the reproductive axis occurs when the loss of weight determines a consistent loss of body fat [42, 43]. In the early stages of dieting or undernutrition or excessive energy consumption, some changes occurring as adaptive response activate the impairment of the reproductive axis as a defensive system, and the more the metabolic defect is, the more intense the negative action becomes (probably) at the hypothalamic level, triggering a greater suppression of the HPG axis [18, 44]. Among the metabolic and energetic signals that act as triggers of this defensive hypothalamic behavior, there are both the insulin and fT3 plasma levels [39, 45, 46]. Any kind of reduced availability of glucose due to excessive consumption and/or decreased acquisition induces hypoinsulinemia that for sure induces specific neuroendocrine effects at the hypothalamic levels, opposite to what happens in case of the compensatory hyperinsulinemia, typical in PCOS [45]. Low levels of fT3 are classically defined as "low T3 syndrome," and this occurs when the reduction of the use of energy for heating purposes is essential. Higher amounts of the biologically inactive reverse-T3 (rT3) are synthesized from peripheral fT4 deiodation, without any change on the feedback signal driving TSH and thyroid hormone synthesis and secretion [39, 40]. In fact, TSH plasma levels are unchanged in patients with FHA.

All such clinical and endocrine data in humans are enforced by a lot of observations in primates in which dieting induces a lot of specific central changes. Just after 1 day of fasting, monkeys show a decrease in the gonadotropin pulsatile secretion with the reduction of LH, FSH, and gonadal steroid secretions [47]. Fasting induces the suppression of the GnRH-induced gonadotropin release, rather than a decrease in pituitary responsiveness to endogenous GnRH [47]. Similar results were observed in humans [48], and in patients with FHA, LH more than FSH seems to be more sensitive to the hypothalamic impairment, since only LH plasma levels are significantly reduced [25]. These data have also enforced the possible existence of an additional system(s) modulating FSH but not LH episodic release from pituitary gland in humans [49, 50].

5.7   Resolution of FHA

FHA is a reversible condition that resolves when metabolic, physical, and psychologic conditions improve. At the basis of the resolution, there is the overlapping of the abovementioned factors, first of all the metabolic factor connected with a positive energy balance where feeding is improved together with a reduced energy consumption, that is, reduced physical activity [51]. The real problem is that such recovery might take several months up to years. A study on the prognosis of FHA reported that the recovery takes place in 7–9 years and the predicting factors are the increase of BMI and the lowering of cortisol plasma levels [52]. Among the elements that might anticipate the recovery, there is the slow elevation of the estradiol plasma levels that anticipates the reduction of the cortisolemia [53]. Such concept is, at least in part, sustained by the recent report on the effects of very low doses of estradiol in FHA patients that showed a specific increase of baseline LH plasma levels and of GnRH-induced LH release [54]. It is of interest to point out that such integrative treatment with hyper-low doses of estradiol was effective in restoring the cortisol response to naloxone infusion though menstrual function is not yet reactivated [54]. Such data support the fact that also minimal changes in estrogenic milieu, both from ovaries and from extraglandular origin, i.e., fat tissue if redeposited, might be a putative positive trigger of the restart of the hypothalamic pathways of the reproductive axis [54].

It is important to remember that FHA classically might show several other symptoms other than that of the amenorrheic condition, such as severe bradycardia, hypotension, orthostasis and/or electrolyte imbalance, osteopenia, and osteoporosis. All these are conditions that need to be recognized and assessed if present so that to define specific medical management [51, 55]. Since FHA is mainly caused by a combination of factors including low weight, excessive exercise, poor nutritional intake, and stress, a multidisciplinary approach is the only beneficial one that has to be applied.

Obviously, restoring a close-to-normal body weight and/or fat mass with a consistent reduction in exercise intensity, restoration of menstrual bleeding may be possible as a sign of a minimum adequate estrogenization of the endometrium having clear that ovulation might not be occurring properly. A high frequency of inadequate luteal phase (low progesterone plasma levels and/or short luteal phases) usually occurs during the first menstrual cycles [56], with a higher ovulating rate being possible with the passing of time and with the maintenance of a proper lifestyle. One of the main targets is the acquisition of a stable body weight, the closer to and possibly higher than the one at which menstruation disappeared. Many patients with FHA have signs of disordered eating or an incipient eating disorder [57, 58] that should be treated with a psychological support so that to change the negative eating habits. In the case of athletes, being difficult to reduce the physical activity and training, a specific psychological support as well as a determinant change in the nutrients and in the quality and amount of food becomes relevant. In those with a formally diagnosed eating disorder, such as AN or bulimia nervosa, referral to specialists in eating disorders is recommended to enable these patients to be appropriately treated by a multidisciplinary team, including psychiatrists.

5.8 Conclusive Remarks

FHA is a classic physiopathological condition that occurs whenever there is the combination of exaggerated physical activity with abnormal feeding and stressful conditions. FHA does not solely occur in athletes or with excessive training. In fact, it may occur also due to stressors acting on the everyday lifestyle. Adolescents and young women should be monitored by family doctors as well as by gynecologists since body weight loss is one of the main physical signs that anticipate the amenorrheic condition.

References

1. Olive DL. Exercise and fertility: an update. Curr Opin Obstet Gynecol. 2010;22(4):259–63.
2. Russell JB, Mitchell D, Musey PI, Collins DC. The relationship of exercise to anovulatory cycles in female athletes: hormonal and physical characteristics. Obstet Gynecol. 1984;63(4):452–6.
3. Otis CL, Drinkwater B, Johnson M, Loucks A, Wilmore J. American College of Sports Medicine position stand. The female athlete triad. Med Sci Sports Exerc. 1997;29(5):i–ix.
4. Rich-Edwards JW, Spiegelman D, Garland M, et al. Physical activity, body mass index, and ovulatory disorder infertility. Epidemiology. 2002;13(2):184–90.
5. Gudmundsdottir SL, Flanders WD, Augestad LB. Physical activity and fertility in women: the North-Trondelag Health Study. Hum Reprod. 2009;24(12):3196–204.
6. Skorseth P, Segovia N, Hastings K, Kraus E. Prevalence of female athlete triad risk factors and iron supplementation among high school distance runners: results from a Triad Risk Screening Toll. Orthop J Sports Med. 2020;8(10):2325967120959725. https://doi.org/10.1177/2325967120959725.
7. (Otis CL, Drinkwater B, Johnson M, et al. American College of Sports Medicine position stand: the female athlete triad. Med Sci Sports Exerc. 2007;39(10):1867–82.) Nattiv A, Loucks AB, Manore MM, Sanborn CF, Sundgot-Borgen J, Warren MP, et al. American College of Sports Medicine position stand. The female athlete triad. Med Sci Sports Exerc. 2007;39(10):1867–82.
8. De Souza MJ, Nattiv A, Joy E, et al. 2014 female athlete triad coalition consensus statement on treatment and return to play of the female athlete triad: 1st International Conference held in San Francisco, California, May 2012 and 2nd International Conference held in Indianapolis, Indiana, May 2013. Br J Sports Med. 2014;48(4):289.
9. Christo K, Prabhakaran R, Lamparello B, et al. Bone metabolism in adolescent athletes with amenorrhea, athletes with eumenorrhea, and control subjects. Pediatrics. 2008;121(6):1127–36.
10. Parks RB, Hetzel SJ, Brooks MA. Iron deficiency and anemia among collegiate athletes: a retrospective chart review. Med Sci Sports Exerc. 2017;49(8):1711–5.
11. Loucks AB. Physical health of the female athlete: observations, effects, and causes of reproductive disorders. Can J Appl Physiol Rev Can Physiol Appl. 2001;26(Suppl):S179–85.
12. Frisch RE, Hall GM, Aoki TT, et al. Metabolic, endocrine, and reproductive changes of a woman channel swimmer. Metabolism. 1984;33(12):1106–11.
13. De Souza MJ, Miller BE, Loucks AB, et al. High frequency of luteal phase deficiency and anovulation in recreational women runners: blunted elevation in follicle-stimulating hormone observed during luteal-follicular transition. J Clin Endocrinol Metab. 1998;83(12):4220–32.
14. Genazzani AD, Gastaldi M, Volpe A, Petraglia F, Genazzani AR. Spontaneous episodic release of adenohypophyseal hormones in hypothalamic amenorrhea. Gynecol Endocrinol. 1995;9(4):325–34.
15. Genazzani AD, Petraglia F, Volpe A, Genazzani AR. Hypothalamic amenorrhea: neuroendocrine mechanisms/stress-induced anomalies. Assist Reprod Technol. 1997;9:1–13.
16. Genazzani AD, Chierchia E, Santagni S, Rattighieri E, Farinetti A, Lanzoni C. Hypothalamic amenorrhea: from diagnosis to therapeutical approach. Ann Endocrinol. 2010;71(3):163–9.
17. Genazzani AD, Despini G, Bonacini R, Prati A. Functional hypothalamic amenorrhea as stress induced defensive system. In: Sultan ARC, Genazzani AR, editors. Frontiers in gynecological endocrinology, ISGE series, vol. 4. Switzerland: Springer Int Publ; 2017. p. 111–8.
18. Rivier C, Rivier J, Vale W. Stress-induced inhibition of reproductive functions: role of endogenous corticotropin-releasing factor. Science. 1986;231:607–9.
19. Petraglia F, Sutton S, Vale W, Plotsky P. Corticotropin-releasing factor decreases plasma luteinizing hormone levels in female rats by inhibiting gonadotropin-releasing hormone release into hypophysial-portal circulation. Endocrinology. 1987;120(3):1083–8.
20. Genazzani AD, Petraglia F, Volpogni C, D'Ambrogio G, Facchinetti F, Genazzani AR. FSH secretory pattern and degree of concordance with LH in amenorrheic, fertile, and postmenopausal women. Am J Physiol. 1993;264(5 Pt 1):E776–81.

21. Petraglia F, Vale W, Rivier C. Opioids act centrally to modulate stress-induced decrease in luteinizing hormone in the rat. Endocrinology. 1986;119(6):2445–50.
22. Ringstrom SJ, Suter D, D'Agostino J, Hoestler JP, Scwartz NB. Effects of glucocorticoids on the hypothalamic-pituitary-gonadal axis. In: Genazzani AR, Nappi G, Petraglia F, Martignoni E, editors. Stress and related disorders from adaptation to dysfunction. Carnforth: Parthenon Publ; 1991. p. 297–305.
23. Cannavò S, Curtò L, Trimarchi F. Exercise-related female reproductive dysfunction. J Endocrinol Invest. 2001;24(10):823–32.
24. American Psychiatric Association. Diagnostic and statistical manual of mental disorders. 4th ed. Washington, DC: American Psychiatric Association; 1995.
25. Genazzani AD, Petraglia F, Fabbri G, Monzani A, Montanini V, Genazzani AR. Evidence of luteinizing hormone secretion in hypothalamic amenorrhea associated with weight loss. Fertil Steril. 1990;54(2):222–6.
26. Vigersky RA, Andersen AE, Thompson RH, Loriaux DL. Hypothalamic dysfunction in secondary amenorrhea associated with simple weight loss. N Engl J Med. 1977;297:1141–5.
27. Berga SL, Mortola SF, Girton L, Suh B, Laughlin G, Pham P, Yen SSC. Neuroendocrine aberrations in women with functional hypothalamic amenorrhea. J Clin Endocrinol Metab. 1989;68(2):301–8.
28. Khoury SA, Reame NE, Kelch RP, Marschall JC. Diurnal patterns of pulsatile luteinizing hormone secretion in hypothalamic amenorrhea: reproducibility and responses to opiate blockade and an alpha2-adrenergic agonist. J Clin Endocrinol Metab. 1987;64(4):755–62.
29. Petraglia F, D'Ambrogio G, Comitini G, Facchinetti F, Volpe A, Genazzani AR. Impairment of opioid control of luteinizing hormone secretion in menstrual disorders. Fertil Steril. 1985;43(4):535–40.
30. Quigley ME, Yen SS. The role of endogenous opiates in LH secretion during the menstrual cycle. J Clin Endocrinol Metab. 1980;51(1):179–81.
31. Lightman SL, Jacobs HS, Maguire AK, McGarrick G, Jeffcoate SL. Constancy of opioid control of luteinizing hormone in different pathophysiological states. J Clin Endocrinol Metab. 1981;52(6):1260–3.
32. Veldhuis JD, Kulin HE, Warner BA, Santner SJ. Responsiveness of gonadotropin secretion to infusion of an opiate-receptor antagonist in hypogonadotropic individuals. J Clin Endocrinol Metab. 1982;55(4):649–53.
33. Remorgida V, Venturini PL, Anserini P, Salerno E, De Cecco L. Naltrexone in functional hypothalamic amenorrhea and in the normal luteal phase. Obstet Gynecol. 1990;76(6):1115–20.
34. Melis GB, Paoletti AM, Gambacciani M, Mais V, Fioretti P. Evidence that estrogens inhibit LH secretion through opioids in postmenopausal women using naloxone. Neuroendocrinology. 1984;39(1):60–3.
35. Snowden UE, Khan-Dawood SF, Dawood MY. The effect of naloxone on endogenous opioid regulation of pituitary gonadotropins and prolactin during the menstrual cycle. J Clin Endocrinol Metab. 1984;59(2):298–302.
36. Petraglia F, Panerai AE, Rivier C, Cocchi D, Genazzani AR. Opioid control of gonadotropin secretion. In: Genazzani AR, Montemagno U, Nappi C, Petraglia F, editors. Brain and female reproductive function. Carnforth: The Parthenon Publishing Group; 1988. p. 65–72.
37. Yen SSC. Opiates and reproduction: studies in women. In: Delitala G, editor. Opioid modulation of endocrine function. New York: Raven Press; 1984. p. 191–9.
38. Kalra SP, Kalra PS. Neural regulation of luteinizing hormone secretion in the rat. Endocr Rev. 1983;4(4):311–51.
39. Genazzani AD, Strucchi C, Malavasi B, Tortolani F, Vecchi F, Luisi S, Petraglia F. Effects of cyproheptadine clorhydrate, a serotonin receptor antagonist, on endocrine parameters in weight-loss related amenorrhea. Gynecol Endocrinol. 2001;15(4):279–85.
40. Fourman LT, Fazeli PK. Neuroendocrine causes of amenorrhea—an update. J Clin Endocrinol Metab. 2015;100(3):812–24.
41. Frisch RE, McArthur JW. Menstrual cycles: fatness as a determinant of minimum weight for height necessary for their maintenance or onset. Science. 1974;185:949–51.

42. Frisch RE. Body fat, puberty and fertility. Biol Rev Camb Philos Soc. 1984;59(2):161–88.
43. Reid RL, Van Vugt DA. Weight-related changes in reproductive function. Fertil Steril. 1987;48(6):905–13.
44. Facchinetti F, Fava M, Fioroni L, Genazzani AD, Genazzani AR. Stressful life events and affective disorders inhibit pulsatile LH secretion in hypothalamic amenorrhea. Psychoneuroendocrinology. 1993;18(5–6):397–404.
45. Genazzani AD, Podfigurna A, Szeliga A, Meczekalski B. Kisspeptin in female reproduction: from physiology to pathophysiology. Gynecol Reprod Endocrinol Metab. 2021;2:148–55.
46. Genazzani AD, Tomatis V, Manzo A, Ressa F, Caroli M, Piccinini M, Ambrosetti F, Arnesano M, Despini G, Meczekalski B. Treatment with carnitines, L-arginine and N-acetyl cysteine in patients affected by functional hypothalamic amenorrhea (FHA) induces hormonal and metabolic changes. Eur Gynecol Obstet. 2020;2(4):239–45.
47. Cameron JL, Nosbich C. Suppression of pulsatile luteinizing hormone and testosterone secretion during short term food restriction in the adult male rhesus monkey (Macaca Mulatta). Endocrinology. 1991;128(3):1532–40.
48. Cameron JL, Weltzin T, McConaha C, Helmreich DL, Kaye WH. Slowing of pulsatile luteinizing hormone secretion in men after forty-eight hours of fasting. J Clin Endocrinol Metab. 1991;73(1):35–41.
49. Genazzani AD, Petraglia F, Gastaldi M, Volpogni C, Gamba O, Massolo F, Genazzani AR. Evidence suggesting an additional control mechanism regulating episodic secretion of luteinizing hormone and follicle stimulating hormone in pre-pubertal children and postmenopausal women. Hum Reprod. 1994;9(10):1807–12.
50. Genazzani AD, Massolo F, Ferrari E, Gandolfi A, Petraglia F, Genazzani AR. Long-term GnRH-agonist administration revealed a GnRH-independent mechanism stimulating FSH discharge in humans. Eur J Endocrinol. 1996;134(1):77–83.
51. Roberts RE, Farahani L, Webber L, Jayasena C. Current understanding of hypothalamic amenorrhoea. Ther Adv Endocrinol Metab. 2020;11:204201882094585. https://doi.org/10.1177/2042018820945854.
52. Falsetti L, Gambera A, Barbetti L, et al. Long-term follow-up of functional hypothalamic amenorrhea and prognostic factors. J Clin Endocrinol Metab. 2002;87(2):500–5.
53. Kondoh Y, Uemura T, Murase M, et al. A longitudinal study of disturbances of the hypothalamic-pituitary-adrenal axis in women with progestin-negative functional hypothalamic amenorrhea. Fertil Steril. 2001;76(4):748–52.
54. Genazzani AD, Despini G, Prati A, Manzo A, Petrillo T, Tomatis V, Giannini A, Simoncini T. Administration of very low doses of estradiol modulates the LH response to a GnRH bolus and the LH and cortisol responses to naloxone infusion in patients with functional hypothalamic amenorrhea (FHA): a pilot study. Endocrines. 2020;1(1):35–45.
55. Society for Adolescent Health and Medicine, Golden NH, Katzman DK, et al. Position paper of the society for adolescent health and medicine: medical management of restrictive eating disorders in adolescents and young adults. J Adolesc Health. 2015;56(1):121–5.
56. Schweiger U. Menstrual function and luteal-phase deficiency in relation to weight changes and dieting. Clin Obstet Gynecol. 1991;34(1):191–7.
57. Berga SL, Marcus MD, Loucks TL, et al. Recovery of ovarian activity in women with functional hypothalamic amenorrhea who were treated with cognitive behavior therapy. Fertil Steril. 2003;80(4):976–81.
58. Michopoulos V, Mancini F, Loucks TL, et al. Neuroendocrine recovery initiated by cognitive behavioral therapy in women with functional hypothalamic amenorrhea: a randomized, controlled trial. Fertil Steril. 2013;99(7):2084–2091.e1.

Sexual Dysfunction in Functional Hypothalamic Amenorrhea

6

Rossella Nappi, Federica Barbagallo, David Bosoni,
Laura Cucinella, Giulia Stincardini, Alessandra Righi,
Manuela Piccinino, Roberta Rossini, and Lara Tiranini

6.1 Introduction

The menstrual cycle should be considered a "vital sign" of overall health and, therefore, many gynecological conditions have an impact on sexual health, including functional hypothalamic amenorrhea (FHA) [1]. However, the involvement of biomedical variables is strongly modulated by psychosocial factors, and only a unified view allows an individualized approach to female sexual dysfunction (FSD). Indeed, FSD is a term used to describe various sexual problems with overlapping organic, intrapersonal, and interpersonal etiologies within the sociocultural context. Any phase of the sexual response cycle may be affected, preventing the individual or the couple from experiencing satisfactory sexual behavior [2]. FSD manifests as chronic sexual symptoms related to sexual pain and the three phases of the sexual response cycle: desire, arousal, and orgasm [2].

Hypothalamic amenorrhea (HA) is a clinical entity very common in women of reproductive age accounting for approximately 30% of cases of secondary amenorrhea [3]. The nonorganic reversible form, named FHA, is characterized by a multitude of neuroendocrine alterations attached to anovulation [4] possibly affecting

R. Nappi (✉) · D. Bosoni · L. Cucinella · G. Stincardini · A. Righi · L. Tiranini
Department of Clinical, Surgical, Diagnostic and Pediatric Sciences, University of Pavia, Pavia, Italy

Research Center for Reproductive Medicine, Gynecological Endocrinology and Menopause, IRCCS San Matteo Foundation, Pavia, Italy

F. Barbagallo
Department of Clinical and Experimental Medicine, University of Catania, Catania, Italy

M. Piccinino · R. Rossini
Department of Clinical, Surgical, Diagnostic and Pediatric Sciences, University of Pavia, Pavia, Italy

© International Society of Gynecological Endocrinology 2023   77
A. R. Genazzani et al. (eds.), *Amenorrhea*, ISGE Series,
https://doi.org/10.1007/978-3-031-22378-5_6

sexual function and behavior. Moreover, risk factors or stressors linked to the development of FHA [5] may equally influence the occurrence of FSD.

Interestingly, two subsequent consensus publications of the International Society of Sexual Medicine recognized the potential impact of FHA on sexuality but outlined the paucity of research on this topic [6, 7].

Here, we will briefly summarize available data on sexuality in women with FHA and we will speculate on potential areas for further investigation.

6.2   Sexual Function and FHA: Modulation of the Neuroendocrine System

It is biologically plausible that sexuality may be impaired in women with FHA because of the peculiar neuroendocrine substrate characterizing these patients [4, 8]. First of all, the suppression of the pulsatile release of gonadotropin-releasing hormone (GnRH) from the hypothalamus impairs the pulsatile release of luteinizing hormone (LH) leading to hypoestrogenism as a result of the absence of growing follicles [4]. The role of estrogens in sexual function is vital acting both within the central nervous system (CNS) and peripheral tissues [9] with clinical implications on breast and vaginal atrophy and manifestation of dyspareunia [10]. In addition, HA is listed among the potential causes of low testosterone due to anovulation, possibly leading to hypoactive sexual desire disorder (HSDD) [11] because of the crucial role of testosterone in modulating CNS areas involved in the long-term control of the central motivational state [12]. Hypoandrogenism may also contribute to the clinical manifestation of sexual symptoms associated with genital involution and poor responsiveness [13]. However, few controversial data are available in women with HA [14, 15], and this condition does not represent an indication for the use of testosterone treatment in the last clinical practice guideline released by the International Society for the Study of Women's Sexual Health (ISSWSH) [16], in line with the Global Consensus Position Statement on the Use of Testosterone Therapy for Women [17]. An early study [14] explored the possibility that impaired sexual function may result from reduced levels of testosterone in subjects with secondary amenorrhea of hypothalamic origin diagnosed according to the presence of risk factors (i.e., weight loss before the onset of amenorrhea, low body weight, strenuous exercise, and vegetarianism). Eight women with HA associated with these particular lifestyles demonstrated impaired sexual function and significantly lower ($p < .03$) circulating testosterone levels (mean ± SEM: 0.84 ± 0.07) as compared with eight normally menstruating women (mean ± SEM: 1.38 ± 0.13). Interestingly, in the experimental setting, women with HA were asked to produce erotic fantasies demonstrating a reduced capacity for sexual fantasizing, less subjective sexual excitement, and less vaginal vasocongestion (vaginal pulse amplitude) with respect to healthy women. Treatment with testosterone undecanoate (40 mg) increased vaginal vasocongestion in women with HA without affecting the subjective sexual experience in response to the exposure to an erotic movie [14]. Apart from exploring testosterone levels in women with HA, this study is important because it formed the basis for understanding that a comprehensive assessment of arousal concerns in women should include both objective assessment of genital arousal and subjective assessment of mental engagement during sexual activity [18]. Another study [15] measured both testosterone and dehydroepiandrosterone sulfate (DHEAS), a pro-hormone that is converted endogenously to androgens and estrogens, in women with anorexia nervosa and normal-weight women with HA. Testosterone and DHEAS levels were superimposable in normal-weight women with HA and healthy controls, whereas they were significantly reduced in women with an overt restrictive eating disorder [15]. In spite of the controversies in linking levels of androgens and sexual function [19] that apply to many gynecological conditions, including polycystic ovary syndrome (PCOS), contraceptive use, and premature menopause [20–22], the potential role of androgens in modulating sexual response deserves further well-conducted studies in different phenotypes of women with FHA [5], especially in those with an ovarian PCOS morphology [23]. Of note, in a cross-sectional Australian study in women aged 18–39 years, a modest association was evident between androgens and sexual function [24], suggesting the need of more in-depth studies to characterize subset of patients. Indeed, normal sexual function has been documented in women with low androgen levels across the menstrual cycle [25], but statistical significant signals correlating androgens with sexual desire were found in a subgroup of women aged 25–44 years with no use of systemic hormonal contraception [26].

Other neuroendocrine, neuro-inflammatory, and neurotrophic processes may be involved in the possible link between sexuality and FHA, as well as thyroid and metabolic disorders, but human studies exploring potential mediators are lacking in this population. Whether sexual function relates to individual sensitivity to different kinds of stressors and to their persistence over time, even at subclinical level, is an area deserving further investigation in FHA [4]. Indeed, high levels of chronic stress measured by salivary cortisol have been related to lower levels of genital sexual arousal, but not subjective arousal responses [27], confirming the complexity of investigating discrete domains of sexual function.

6.3   Sexual Function and FHA: The Importance of Mood

Mood disorders may be the result of the neurobiological adaptive responses typically associated with FHA or may constitute a vulnerable background of stress sensitivity [4]. Stressful life events and affective disorders inhibited pulsatile LH secretion in HA [28] and may predispose to behavioral adaptations to cope with stress, including change of eating habits or exercise load [4]. It is conceivable that the high rates of mood disorders consistently documented in women with FHA [29, 30] play a role in the occurrence of FSD. The common link could be the increased activity of hypothalamic-pituitary-adrenal (HPA) axis associated with the impairment of some central pathways (opioids and serotonin) in patients with HA [31]. Indeed, chronic elevation of glucocorticoid hormones (e.g., cortisol) can have adverse effects on brain structure and function contributing to mental illness [32].

Mood changes, depression, and anxiety are common experiences among women who suffer from FSD [33, 34]. The use of a 2-week daily diary approach to examine same-day and temporal relations between affective symptoms and sexual function in a nonclinical sample of young women found that depression-specific anhedonia and sexual desire were closely related [35]. Also, physiological hyperarousal associated with anxiety gave rise to sexual arousal difficulties and vaginal pain, whereas increases in general distress were linked with difficulties achieving orgasm [35].

By using the Italian McCoy Female Sexuality Questionnaire (MFSQ-I) and two validated questionnaires to assess anxiety and depression, Dundon et al. [36] explored the relationship between FHA and FSD and the possible mediating role of mood disorders. Women with FHA ($n = 41$) showed significantly lower scores ($p < .001$) in overall sexual function than control women ($n = 39$), whereas scores on satisfaction with sexual relationship with partner were very similar between the two groups [36]. These data suggested that women with FHA attributed their sexual problems to feelings of inadequacy and low self-esteem, which are common personality characteristics, along with poor flexibility, perfectionism, and need for social approval [37]. Interestingly, only depression offered a significant explanation for the sexual problems experienced by women with FHA, although depression and anxiety were both significantly higher ($p < .001$) as compared to control women. Among the multitude of factors implicated in the functional etiology and maintenance of HA, clinicians should routinely screen also FSD to counsel patients on this important aspect of their quality of life. Therapeutic goals include replacing reproductive hormones to minimize the long-term consequences of estrogen deprivation [1, 4, 5], but inadequate information is available regarding the ability of hormone replacement to ameliorate mood and sexual function. That being so, cognitive behavioral therapy (CBT), an effective method to restore ovarian function in FHA [38] by identifying those relevant metabolic, behavioral, and psychological factors that act as stressors, should provide a strategic plan also for sexual symptoms by means of psychosocial approaches [39].

Whether FSD may precede the onset of FHA is unknown, and longitudinal studies will possibly address this question.

6.4　Sexual Function and FHA: Expanding Our Understanding on the Role of Other Possible Mediators

In the context of the biopsychosocial model, women with FHA and those with FSD share many potential risk factors [2] besides endocrine abnormalities and mood disorders. FSD is common across eating disorder subtypes, and low BMI is associated with loss of libido, sexual anxiety, and avoidance of sexual relationships [40]. In a study exploring the association between physical activity and sexual pain, patients between the ages of 18 and 30 years who were normal or underweight reported the highest risk [41]. In addition, sexual pain was present in more than 50% of physically active women, without a significant impact of weekly energy expenditure from exercise [41]. Sexual functioning was found to be deeply interconnected with the core psychopathology of eating disorders, which includes body image disturbance and deficit of embodiment [42]. Common pathways connect the areas of emotion dysregulation/impulsivity and perfectionism/overcontrol both with eating disorder-specific psychopathology and with different types of sexual impairment [43]. A history of sexual abuse in women with eating disorders may also be present and associated with dissociative experiences during sexual activity or sexual stimulation contributing to FSD [43]. In particular, patients with a history of childhood traumatic experiences or with anxious attachment have been reported to engage in risky sexual behaviors [43]. Interestingly, increased childhood adversity may influence fertility difficulties and menstrual cycle patterns [44]. Compared to women with no adversity, women in the high-adversity group were more likely to experience both infertility and amenorrhea (RR = 2.75, 95% CI 1.45–5.21, and RR = 2.54, 95% CI 1.52–4.25, respectively) [44].

Finally, menstruation is the hallmark of womanhood representing a clear biological sign of reproductive ability [45], which is linked to sexual behavior. The experiences of infertility in women with FHA may contribute to the impairment of sexual function, but data are lacking.

6.5 Conclusions

FHA includes a constellation of neuroendocrine aberrations associated with several stressors with a possible significance in the context of sexual health. It seems mandatory to screen for FSD as part of a comprehensive approach to the quality of life of women with FHA bearing in mind that research is still in its infancy. However, we believe that it will take time to fully understand the contribution of different factors to sexual function and behavior of these patients and only long-term studies investigating several areas of psychosexual well-being early in adolescent development will shed light on the multifaceted etiology of both FHA and FSD. Treatment strategies should always follow the biopsychosocial model, and counselling appears fundamental to address at the same time the numerous concerns contributing to reproductive failure.

References

1. Shufelt CL, Torbati T, Dutra E. Hypothalamic amenorrhea and the long-term health consequences. Semin Reprod Med. 2017;35(3):256–62. https://doi.org/10.1055/s-0037-1603581.
2. Parish SJ, Cottler-Casanova S, Clayton AH, McCabe MP, Coleman E, Reed GM. The evolution of the female sexual disorder/dysfunction definitions, nomenclature, and classifications: a review of DSM, ICSM, ISSWSH, and ICD. Sex Med Rev. 2021;9(1):36–56. https://doi.org/10.1016/j.sxmr.2020.05.001.
3. Reindollar RH, Novak M, Tho SP, McDonough PG. Adult-onset amenorrhea: a study of 262 patients. Am J Obstet Gynecol. 1986;155(3):531–43. https://doi.org/10.1016/0002-9378(86)90274-7.
4. Ruiz-Zambrana A, Berga SL. A clinician's guide to functional hypothalamic amenorrhea. Clin Obstet Gynecol. 2020;63(4):706–19. https://doi.org/10.1097/GRF.0000000000000573.

5. Gordon CM, Ackerman KE, Berga SL, Kaplan JR, Mastorakos G, Misra M, Murad MH, Santoro NF, Warren MP. Functional hypothalamic amenorrhea: an Endocrine Society clinical practice guideline. J Clin Endocrinol Metab. 2017;102(5):1413–39. https://doi.org/10.1210/jc.2017-00131.

6. Wierman ME, Nappi RE, Avis N, Davis SR, Labrie F, Rosner W, Shifren JL. Endocrine aspects of women's sexual function. J Sex Med. 2010;7(1 Pt 2):561–85. https://doi.org/10.1111/j.1743-6109.2009.01629.x.

7. Worsley R, Santoro N, Miller KK, Parish SJ, Davis SR. Hormones and female sexual dysfunction: beyond estrogens and androgens—findings from the Fourth International Consultation on Sexual Medicine. J Sex Med. 2016;13(3):283–90. https://doi.org/10.1016/j.jsxm.2015.12.014.

8. Genazzani AD, Chierchia E, Santagni S, Rattighieri E, Farinetti A, Lanzoni C. Hypothalamic amenorrhea: from diagnosis to therapeutical approach. Ann Endocrinol (Paris). 2010;71(3):163–9. https://doi.org/10.1016/j.ando.2010.02.006.

9. Nappi RE, Polatti F. The use of estrogen therapy in women's sexual functioning (CME). J Sex Med. 2009;6(3):603–16; quiz 618–9. https://doi.org/10.1111/j.1743-6109.2008.01198.x.

10. Huhmann K. Menses requires energy: a review of how disordered eating, excessive exercise, and high stress lead to menstrual irregularities. Clin Ther. 2020;42(3):401–7. https://doi.org/10.1016/j.clinthera.2020.01.016.

11. Davis SR, Worsley R, Miller KK, Parish SJ, Santoro N. Androgens and female sexual function and dysfunction—findings from the Fourth International Consultation of Sexual Medicine. J Sex Med. 2016;13(2):168–78. https://doi.org/10.1016/j.jsxm.2015.12.033.

12. Ågmo A, Laan E. Sexual incentive motivation, sexual behavior, and general arousal: do rats and humans tell the same story? Neurosci Biobehav Rev. 2022;135:104595. https://doi.org/10.1016/j.neubiorev.2022.104595.

13. Simon JA, Goldstein I, Kim NN, Davis SR, Kellogg-Spadt S, Lowenstein L, Pinkerton JV, Stuenkel CA, Traish AM, Archer DF, Bachmann G, Goldstein AT, Nappi RE, Vignozzi L. The role of androgens in the treatment of genitourinary syndrome of menopause (GSM): International Society for the Study of Women's Sexual Health (ISSWSH) expert consensus panel review. Menopause. 2018;25(7):837–47. https://doi.org/10.1097/GME.0000000000001138.

14. Tuiten A, Laan E, Panhuysen G, Everaerd W, de Haan E, Koppeschaar H, Vroon P. Discrepancies between genital responses and subjective sexual function during testosterone substitution in women with hypothalamic amenorrhea. Psychosom Med. 1996;58(3):234–41. https://doi.org/10.1097/00006842-199605000-00007.

15. Miller KK, Lawson EA, Mathur V, Wexler TL, Meenaghan E, Misra M, Herzog DB, Klibanski A. Androgens in women with anorexia nervosa and normal-weight women with hypothalamic amenorrhea. J Clin Endocrinol Metab. 2007;92(4):1334–9. https://doi.org/10.1210/jc.2006-2501.

16. Parish SJ, Simon JA, Davis SR, Giraldi A, Goldstein I, Goldstein SW, Kim NN, Kingsberg SA, Morgentaler A, Nappi RE, Park K, Stuenkel CA, Traish AM, Vignozzi L. International Society for the Study of Women's Sexual Health clinical practice guideline for the use of systemic testosterone for hypoactive sexual desire disorder in women. J Womens Health (Larchmt). 2021;30(4):474–91. https://doi.org/10.1089/jwh.2021.29037.

17. Davis SR, Baber R, Panay N, Bitzer J, Perez SC, Islam RM, Kaunitz AM, Kingsberg SA, Lambrinoudaki I, Liu J, Parish SJ, Pinkerton J, Rymer J, Simon JA, Vignozzi L, Wierman ME. Global consensus position statement on the use of testosterone therapy for women. J Clin Endocrinol Metab. 2019;104(10):4660–6. https://doi.org/10.1210/jc.2019-01603.

18. Meston CM, Stanton AM. Understanding sexual arousal and subjective-genital arousal desynchrony in women. Nat Rev Urol. 2019;16(2):107–20. https://doi.org/10.1038/s41585-018-0142-6.

19. Nappi RE. To be or not to be in sexual desire: the androgen dilemma. Climacteric. 2015;18(5):672–4. https://doi.org/10.3109/13697137.2015.1064268.

20. Nappi RE, Tiranini L. Polycystic ovary syndrome and sexuality. Gynecol Endocrinol. 2022;38(7):535–6. https://doi.org/10.1080/09513590.2022.2089109.

21. Nappi RE, Tiranini L. "50 Shades of sex" under hormonal contraception. Gynecol Endocrinol. 2020;36(9):753–4. https://doi.org/10.1080/09513590.2020.1811847.

22. Nappi RE, Cucinella L, Martini E, Rossi M, Tiranini L, Martella S, Bosoni D, Cassani C. Sexuality in premature ovarian insufficiency. Climacteric. 2019;22(3):289–95. https://doi.org/10.1080/13697137.2019.1575356.

23. Phylactou M, Clarke SA, Patel B, Baggaley C, Jayasena CN, Kelsey TW, Comninos AN, Dhillo WS, Abbara A. Clinical and biochemical discriminants between functional hypothalamic amenorrhoea (FHA) and polycystic ovary syndrome (PCOS). Clin Endocrinol (Oxf). 2021;95(2):239–52. https://doi.org/10.1111/cen.14402.

24. Zheng J, Islam RM, Skiba MA, Bell RJ, Davis SR. Associations between androgens and sexual function in premenopausal women: a cross-sectional study. Lancet Diabetes Endocrinol. 2020;8(8):693–702. https://doi.org/10.1016/S2213-8587(20)30239-4.

25. Salonia A, Pontillo M, Nappi RE, Zanni G, Fabbri F, Scavini M, Daverio R, Gallina A, Rigatti P, Bosi E, Bonini PA, Montorsi F. Menstrual cycle-related changes in circulating androgens in healthy women with self-reported normal sexual function. J Sex Med. 2008;5:854–63.

26. Wåhlin-Jacobsen S, Pedersen AT, Kristensen E, Laessøe NC, Lundqvist M, Cohen AS, Hougaard DM, Giraldi A. Is there a correlation between androgens and sexual desire in women? J Sex Med. 2015;12(2):358–73. https://doi.org/10.1111/jsm.12774.

27. Hamilton LD, Meston CM. Chronic stress and sexual function in women. J Sex Med. 2013;10(10):2443–54. https://doi.org/10.1111/jsm.12249.

28. Facchinetti F, Fava M, Fioroni L, Genazzani AD, Genazzani AR. Stressful life events and affective disorders inhibit pulsatile LH secretion in hypothalamic amenorrhea. Psychoneuroendocrinology. 1993;18(5–6):397–404. https://doi.org/10.1016/0306-4530(93)90014-c.

29. Marcus MD, Loucks TL, Berga SL. Psychological correlates of functional hypothalamic amenorrhea. Fertil Steril. 2001;76(2):310–6. https://doi.org/10.1016/s0015-0282(01)01921-5.

30. Nappi RE, Facchinetti F. Psychoneuroendocrine correlates of secondary amenorrhea. Arch Womens Ment Health. 2003;6(2):83–9. https://doi.org/10.1007/s00737-002-0152-4.

31. Nappi RE, Petraglia F, Genazzani AD, D'Ambrogio G, Zara C, Genazzani AR. Hypothalamic amenorrhea: evidence for a central derangement of hypothalamic-pituitary-adrenal cortex axis activity. Fertil Steril. 1993;59(3):571–6.

32. McEwen BS, Bowles NP, Gray JD, Hill MN, Hunter RG, Karatsoreos IN, Nasca C. Mechanisms of stress in the brain. Nat Neurosci. 2015;18(10):1353–63. https://doi.org/10.1038/nn.4086.

33. Shifren JL, Monz BU, Russo PA, Segreti A, Johannes CB. Sexual problems and distress in United States women: prevalence and correlates. Obstet Gynecol. 2008;112(5):970–8. https://doi.org/10.1097/AOG.0b013e3181898cdb.

34. Basson R, Gilks T. Women's sexual dysfunction associated with psychiatric disorders and their treatment. Womens Health (Lond). 2018;14:1745506518762664. https://doi.org/10.1177/1745506518762664.

35. Kalmbach DA, Kingsberg SA, Ciesla JA. How changes in depression and anxiety symptoms correspond to variations in female sexual response in a nonclinical sample of young women: a daily diary study. J Sex Med. 2014;11(12):2915–27. https://doi.org/10.1111/jsm.12692.

36. Dundon CM, Rellini AH, Tonani S, Santamaria V, Nappi R. Mood disorders and sexual functioning in women with functional hypothalamic amenorrhea. Fertil Steril. 2010;94(6):2239–43. https://doi.org/10.1016/j.fertnstert.2010.01.012.

37. Giles DE, Berga SL. Cognitive and psychiatric correlates of functional hypothalamic amenorrhea: a controlled comparison. Fertil Steril. 1993;60(3):486–92.

38. Berga SL, Marcus MD, Loucks TL, Hlastala S, Ringham R, Krohn MA. Recovery of ovarian activity in women with functional hypothalamic amenorrhea who were treated with cognitive behavior therapy. Fertil Steril. 2003;80(4):976–81. https://doi.org/10.1016/s0015-0282(03)01124-5.

39. Kingsberg SA, Althof S, Simon JA, Bradford A, Bitzer J, Carvalho J, Flynn KE, Nappi RE, Reese JB, Rezaee RL, Schover L, Shifrin JL. Female sexual dysfunction-medical and psychological treatments, committee 14. J Sex Med. 2017;14(12):1463–91. https://doi.org/10.1016/j.jsxm.2017.05.018.

40. Pinheiro AP, Raney TJ, Thornton LM, Fichter MM, Berrettini WH, Goldman D, Halmi KA, Kaplan AS, Strober M, Treasure J, Woodside DB, Kaye WH, Bulik CM. Sexual functioning

in women with eating disorders. Int J Eat Disord. 2010;43(2):123–9. https://doi.org/10.1002/eat.20671.

41. Fergus KB, Cohen AJ, Cedars BE, Rowen TS, Patino G, Breyer BN. Risk factors for sexual pain among physically active women. Sex Med. 2020;8(3):501–9. https://doi.org/10.1016/j.esxm.2020.03.007.

42. Castellini G, Rossi E, Ricca V. The relationship between eating disorder psychopathology and sexuality: etiological factors and implications for treatment. Curr Opin Psychiatry. 2020;33(6):554–61. https://doi.org/10.1097/YCO.0000000000000646.

43. Castellini G, Rossi E, Ricca V. Are there common pathways for eating disorders and female sexual dysfunction? J Sex Med. 2022;19(1):8–11. https://doi.org/10.1016/j.jsxm.2021.10.006.

44. Jacobs MB, Boynton-Jarrett RD, Harville EW. Adverse childhood event experiences, fertility difficulties and menstrual cycle characteristics. J Psychosom Obstet Gynaecol. 2015;36(2):46–57. https://doi.org/10.3109/0167482X.2015.1026892.

45. Critchley HOD, Babayev E, Bulun SE, Clark S, Garcia-Grau I, Gregersen PK, Kilcoyne A, Kim JJ, Lavender M, Marsh EE, Matteson KA, Maybin JA, Metz CN, Moreno I, Silk K, Sommer M, Simon C, Tariyal R, Taylor HS, Wagner GP, Griffith LG. Menstruation: science and society. Am J Obstet Gynecol. 2020;223(5):624–64. https://doi.org/10.1016/j.ajog.2020.06.004.

Endocrine Gland Disorder-Related Amenorrhoea

Diana Jędrzejuk and Andrzej Milewicz

7.1 Introduction

Amenorrhoea is the absence or cessation of menstruation. Amenorrhoea is conventionally divided into primary and secondary amenorrhoea. In this chapter, we focus on secondary amenorrhoea, which means that menstruation starts but then stops. The endocrine gland disorders play a crucial role in menstrual irregularity and in amenorrhoea. The menstrual cycle includes ovarian and endometrial cycles in which the cyclic response to the hormone production from the hypothalamus, pituitary, thyroid as well as adrenals leads to the occurrence of menstrual cycle. We focus on the hormonal changes and results of menstrual disturbances, which have been observed in pituitary, thyroid and adrenal disorders.

7.2 Pituitary Tumours

Pituitary adenomas are the most common reason for hypothalamic-pituitary system disorders, the etiopathogenesis of which is complex and not fully clarified. Adenomas frequently result in hyperpituitarism; hypopituitarism is observed rarely.

D. Jędrzejuk (✉)
Department of Endocrinology, Diabetes and Isotope Therapy, Wrocław Medical University, Wroclaw, Poland
e-mail: diana.jedrzejuk@umw.edu.pl

A. Milewicz
Department of Endocrinology, Diabetes and Isotope Therapy, Wrocław Medical University, Wroclaw, Poland

Medical and Technical Sciences, Karkonosze University of Applied Sciences, Jelenia Góra, Poland
e-mail: andrzej.milewicz@umw.edu.pl

© International Society of Gynecological Endocrinology 2023
A. R. Genazzani et al. (eds.), *Amenorrhea*, ISGE Series,
https://doi.org/10.1007/978-3-031-22378-5_7

Hyperpituitarism is usually accompanied by prolactin (PRL) excessive release due to microadenoma (tumour diameter smaller than 10 mm) or macroadenoma (tumour diameter bigger than 10 mm) presence. Growth hormone (GH) release is observed less frequently.

7.2.1   Hyperprolactinaemia

Hyperprolactinaemia is prolactin excessive release, which physiologically accompanies pregnancy, lactation or physical exertion. Its pathological character is observed in pituitary gland adenoma in patients with hypothalamic pituitary system disorders or liver or kidney failure or as drugs' side effect. Prolactinomas are the most common pituitary tumours, and they constitute up to 40% of all tumours. They prevail more often in females than in males: 30/100,000 vs. 10/100,000.

Hyperprolactinaemia increases hypothalamus endorphin neuron activity, resulting in gonadotropin-releasing hormone (GnRH) pulse impairment [1]. As a consequence, pituitary gonadotropin-luteinising hormone (LH) as well as follicle-stimulating hormone (FSH) release is disturbed, too. In females, the Graafian follicle development as well as ovaries' endocrine activity are inhibited, which provokes oestradiol and progesterone deficiency. In females, hyperprolactinaemia results in galactorrhoea. Corpus luteum insufficiency with preserved ovary oestrogen function may result in mastodynia. The most common symptom of female hyperprolactinaemia is menstrual cycle disturbances. Along with prolactin concentration growth, luteal phase deficiency is observed followed by anovulation, scarce and rare menstruation and absolute amenorrhoea called "secondary amenorrhoea". In 25% of hyperprolactinaemia cases, macroprolactin (big-big prolactin) predominant form is observed, and it is prolactin bound with anti-PRL immunoglobulin G (IgG). In practice, in macroprolactinaemia patients, hyperprolactinaemia with normal ovulation cycle is diagnosed.

Prolactinoma diagnosis is based upon amenorrhoea-galactorrhoea syndrome recognition, increased prolactin concentration (over 150.0 microg/L) definition as well as magnetic resonance imaging (MRI) visualisation of pituitary adenoma. Hyperprolactinaemia of 25.0–150.0 microg/L is a frequent and difficult diagnostic problem of functional or iatrogenic origin. In such cases, the goal of treatment is prolactin concentration normalisation and gonad normal function restoration. As a result, menstruation abnormalities and galactorrhoea regress, libido and fertility are restored and the risk of osteoporosis is limited.

Drugs of choice are dopamine agonists, which not only inhibit PRL secretion but also provoke tumour regression. The oldest (40 years on the stock), the cheapest and the most effective drug is ergot derivative—bromocriptine, applied in doses dependent on PRL level. With available tablets (2.5 mg), administration starts with 2.5 mg daily at night, and after 5 days, the dose is gradually increased by ½ tablet. After next 5 days, it is increased by another ½ tablet up to where therapeutic dose is finally achieved. Therapeutic dose depends on PRL level, and it amounts to 2.5–30.0 mg/24 h due to side effects such as blood pressure orthostatic decrease, nausea, vomiting constipation and drowsiness. As its activity persists for 8–12 h, administration twice a day is recommended.

Another drug is quinagolide, the activity of which persists for 24 h; daily dose is dependent on PRL level and amounts to 75–600 microg/24 h. The risk of side effects is smaller than in the case of bromocriptine. Cabergoline is a drug of the longest duration. It can be administered once or twice a week in a dose dependent on PRL concentration, which is 0.5–3.0 mg per week. It reveals the biggest efficacy and the smallest number of side effects. However, the risk of cardiac valve fibrosis should be taken into account with cabergoline's prolonged administration. This drug application provides prolactin concentration normalisation in 90–95% of patients. In 90% of patients, it provokes tumour size reduction. Operative treatment is indicated in cases of pharmacotherapy intolerance or resistance. Its results depend upon tumour size and location.

7.2.2 Acromegaly

Acromegaly is a chronic disease resulting from growth hormone excessive production and most often, in 99%, it is caused by pituitary adenoma autonomic secretion. Only sporadically, it results from excessive release of growth hormone by neuroendocrine neoplasms. Macroadenomas (diameter bigger than 10 mm) constitute about 80% of all adenomas. Smaller tumours are rare. Majority of tumours (about ¾) are built of somatotropic cells. The remaining ones also release prolactin due to mammotropic cells' presence, and somatotropic and mammotropic mixed form is rather rare. Excessive release of growth hormone results in patient's appearance change such as palms, feet and facial structure enlargement as well as soft tissues. Hyperplasia of bones and internal organs may occur, and many other complications including cardiovascular system are the reason for increased mortality. The possible manifestation on menstrual cycle due to the higher levels of prolactin and oestrogen deficiency was observed in acromegaly. Kaltsas et al.'s [2] study showed that 62% of patients with acromegaly experienced amenorrhoea, 15% had oligomenorrhoea and 4% had polymenorrhoea. Data from the multi-centre acromegaly registry reported that hypogonadism was observed in more than half of the women with acromegaly [3].

Diagnosis of active acromegaly is carried out on the basis of characteristic clinical symptoms and signs, hormonal disturbances as well as presence of pituitary tumour found in MRI. In hormonal diagnosis, if insulin-like growth factor-1 (IGF-1) values are increased, it is recommended to perform an oral glucose tolerance test (OGTT) after administration of 75 g of glucose. The diagnosis is confirmed by an increased IGF-1 concentration and no suppression of GH secretion below 0.4 microg/L (ng/mL) in OGTT. Random GH level below 1.0 microg/L allows the exclusion of active acromegaly [4]. Operative treatment is recommended, but if it does not bring GH concentration and IGF-1 normalisation, somatostatin analogue therapy should be introduced.

7.2.3 Cushing's Disease

Cushing's disease is a hypercortisolaemia condition induced by adrenocorticotropic hormone (ACTH) excessive release (ACTH-dependent Cushing's syndrome). Most often, in 95%, it is caused by ACTH-releasing pituitary isolated adenoma. In about 5% of cases, primary disturbances of hypothalamic corticoliberin or vasopressin release are probably related to corticotropic cell hyperplasia. Besides, Cushing's disease can be a component of multiple endocrine neoplasia type 1 syndrome (MEN1). Clinically, it is characteristic for reddened and round face (moon-shaped face), red skin stretches, neck and corpus fat deposition (central obesity), atrophy of limb muscles, hypertension, diabetes and osteoporosis. In turn, Cushing's syndrome (non-ACTH-dependent Cushing's syndrome) is every hypercortisolaemia condition not provoked by ACTH release and also caused by adrenal carcinoma. In majority of Cushing's disease patients, gonad function abnormalities are observed. Hypercortisolaemia disturbs GnRH release and inhibits gonadotropin secretion. In females, it results in menstruation disturbances (oligomenorrhea, amenorrhea) in 56–80% woman affected by hypercortisolemia and infertility [1]. Menstrual irregularity seems to be most closely related to the level of serum cortisol rather than androgen level [5]. Obviously, increased ACTH release results in increased androgen production and hyperandrogenism favours seborrhoea, acne and hirsutism.

In diagnostics, 1.0 mg dexamethasone application proves to be useful in testing cortisol release inhibition. In physiological conditions, after oral administration of 1.0 mg dexamethasone dose at 11 pm, on the next day, cortisol concentration determined at 8 am is below 1.8 µg/dL (50.0 nmol/L); the Cushing's syndrome is excluded. Besides, increased cortisol concentration determined in 24-h urine collection is also very useful in a diagnostic process.

Surgical treatment of adenocarcinoma is of strategic importance in the course of the whole therapy. Steroidogenesis inhibitors should be applied in hypercortisolaemic patients before the operation. In the case of insufficient effect of the therapy, reoperation is indicated as well as adrenalectomy and radiotherapy subsequently. Inefficacy of surgical treatment may be corrected by applying pasireotide—a new somatostatin analogue, which reveals big affinity to somatostatin receptor fifth type.

7.3   Thyroid Disorders

Thyroid hormones are essential for proper development and differentiation of all cells of the human body. They affect the female reproductive organ; in combination with FSH, triiodothyronine enhances granulose cell proliferation and inhibits granulose cell apoptosis by the protein kinase B pathway. Thyroid hormone receptors are expressed in endometrium [6]. The highest level of expression of thyroid hormone receptors was found in receptive endometrium, and it proved that thyroid hormones influence endometrial function [7]. Transcripts required for thyroid hormone synthesis and metabolism such as thyroid peroxidase, thyroglobulin and 5-deiodinase type 2 were also identified in human endometrium, suggesting possible thyroid hormone production [8]. Expression of TSH and thyroid hormone receptors was revealed in human oocytes in physiological and non-physiological methods, during in vitro fertilisation (IVF) programme, conditions indicating direct thyroid hormone action in human ovaries. Deiodinase-2 and deiodinase-3 transcripts were determined in granulosa cells, suggesting their ability to control local hormone activity through deiodination of T4 to either T3 or, to a lesser extent, reverse T3 [6, 9, 10].

Leukaemia inhibitory factor (LIF) is involved in the embryo implantation process and expressed in the mid-secretory endometrium. TSH significantly upregulates leukaemia inhibitory factor expression in endometrial cell cultures, which suggests a potential role of TSH in the implantation process. For that reason, we can expect reproduction disturbances in case of thyroid disorders [10].

7.3.1 Hypothyroidism

The prevalence of menstrual abnormalities reported is 25–60% in hypothyroid women compared to 10% in euthyroid women. The predominant menstrual disturbance in hypothyroid women described is oligomenorrhoea [11, 12]. Thyroid autoimmunity (TAI) is the most frequent autoimmune disorder in women of childbearing age, and it increases the risk of thyroid dysfunction. The prevalence of TAI is generally estimated at around 10% [13]. In women with elevated anti-thyroperoxidase (ATPO) antibody titres, the relative risk of female infertility is increased [14, 15].

Hypothyroidism may also lead to a diminished LH response, thereby stimulating thyrotropin-releasing hormone (TRH) secretion and increasing serum prolactin levels. As PRL impairs pulsatile secretion of GnRH, this can lead to ovulatory dysfunction [12, 15]. For that reason, in hypothyroidism, we can expect decrease of serum oestradiol and sex hormone-binding globulin (SHBG), increase of PRL and androstenedione as well as impaired GnRH secretion, resulting in menstrual irregularities and anovulation [13]. Clinical symptoms of hypothyroidism are the following: fatigue, increased sensitivity of cold, constipation, dry skin, weight gain, puffy face, muscle weakness, muscle aches, tenderness and stiffness, pain, stiffness or swelling joints, heavier-than-normal or irregular menstrual periods, secondary amenorrhoea, thinning of hair, slowed heart rate, depression and impaired memory.

Diagnosis is based on elevated serum TSH levels over 5.0 mIU/L as well as FT4 lower than 0.7 ng/dL (normal range of TSH 0.5–5.0 mIU/L, FT4 0.7–1.9 microg/dL).

The L-thyroxin is the first-choice therapy, and it proves to be very successful; hormonal changes and menstrual pattern may normalise [16].

7.3.2 Hyperthyroidism

Studies on the prevalence of subfertility in women with hyperthyroidism are limited. Majority of them are uncontrolled, retrospective and small population studies. In contrast to hypothyroidism, increased serum SHBG is characteristic for hyperthyroidism so much that this globulin is used as a test of thyroid function, revealing tissue response to the thyroid hormone. It should be considered when levels of oestradiol and testosterone are interpreted because the total amounts are increased out of proportion to free levels. It has been published that total oestrogen levels may be two- to threefold higher in hyperthyroid women (compared to normal women) [17]. Serum LH and FSH may also be increased; mean LH levels are higher in hyperthyroid women (compared to normal women) [17–19]. It has been published that during the early follicular phase of the menstrual cycle, the LH secretion was increased in hyperthyroid women with GD, whereas the pulsatile characteristics of LH and FSH secretion did not differ in patients when compared to controls [18, 20, 21]. Serum LH levels decrease to normal after a few weeks of treatment with anti-thyroid drugs (ATD) [19]. The mechanism underlying the increase in serum LH in hyperthyroid women is as yet unclear [16].

In prepuberty girls, menstruation has been reported to be delayed [16, 17]. The primary or secondary infertility in 5.8% of hyperthyroid patients has been presented, but other prospective studies have showed the prevalence of suppressed TSH (subclinical or overt hyperthyroidism) in 2.1% compared to 3% in fertile controls [12, 14]. Despite a comparable prevalence of hyperthyroidism, suppressed TSH was more prevalent in antibody-positive compared to antibody-negative patients [14]. Recent data showed a lower prevalence of menstrual abnormalities of about 22% compared to 8% in healthy controls [22]. Clinical symptoms of hyperthyroidism are the following: (1) non-specific symptoms like tachycardia, increased sweating, nervousness, tremor and weight loss and/or (2) specific symptoms like goitre, thyroid ophthalmopathy, pretibial oedema, lower serum TSH (normal range of TSH 0.5–5.0 mIU/L), proximal myopathy, weight loss and increased TRAb titre.

For thyrotoxicosis therapy, propylthiouracil (PTU) or methimazole (MMI) is recommended. However, in the first and second trimesters of pregnancy, PTU and MHI therapies are recommended, respectively [23]. They are also not contraindication to breastfeeding in women treated for hypo- and hyperthyroidism [23].

7.4   Adrenal Gland Disorders

Non-classical congenital adrenal hyperplasia (N-CCAH) is another disorder that may influence the menstrual cycle; the most common manifestations of menstrual disorder in these patients are primary or secondary amenorrhoea and oligomenorrhoea.

7.4.1   Non-classical Congenital Adrenal Hyperplasia Due to 21 Hydroxylase Deficiency

N-CCAH due to 21-hydroxylase deficiency is one of the most common congenital autosomal diseases, and it results from CYP21A2 gene mutation. This abnormality is observed in 1–2% of androgenic females. 21-Hydroxylase deficiency causes cortisol synthesis inhibition, increased ACTH release and increased androgen secretion, and in severe cases, it results in deoxycortisol and aldosterone deficiency. Shortage of cortisol provokes pituitary gland to release increased amounts of ACTH which, in turn, stimulates adrenal glands. 17-Hydroxyprogesterone (17-OHP) is accumulated which, due to 21-hydroxylase block, does not turn into 11-deoxycortisol and cortisol, and progesterone does not turn to 11-deoxycorticosterone. Steroids, the synthesis of which is not disturbed, are accumulated and adrenal androgens [dehydroepiandrosterone (DHEA), dehydroepiandrosterone sulphate (DHEAS), androstenedione and testosterone] are excessively released.

Clinical picture of non-classical and late-onset form of the disease is characteristic for preserving 20–50% of 21-hydroxylase activity and moderate increase of androgen synthesis. In this form of N-CCAH, symptoms develop later; they are diverse and hard to recognise. They may include premature puberty, purulent acne, preterm growth and epiphyseal plate preterm mineralisation, which finally may result in short stature. Non-classical form signs and symptoms are observed in adulthood, and they are diagnosed in females only as they reveal hirsutism, seborrhoea, temporal alopecia, clitoris enlargement, menstruation abnormalities and infertility. The disease increases the risk of metabolic syndrome. During the diagnostic process, apart from the above clinical symptoms, some other specific manifestations should be established. These are increased concentration of 17-OHP over 10.0 ng/mL, increased concentration of androgen ACTH in plasma as well as 17-ketosteroid presence in urine. Concentration of 17-OHP over 10.0 ng/mL after 60 min with ACTH intravenous stimulation confirms diagnosis of non-classical form. Increased levels of DHEA, androstenedione and testosterone are observed as well. In order to avoid the development of polycystic ovary syndrome (PCOS), oral contraceptives are administered to females with non-classical form of congenital adrenal cortex hyperplasia. In case of strong androgenisation, spironolactone or flutamide is applied. The therapy should be monitoring of 17-OHP concentration in serum. In case of females in their reproductive period who do not use contraceptives or in those during pregnancy, dexamethasone should be replaced with hydrocortisone. Dexamethasone penetrates placenta, and it can adversely affect the functioning of hypothalamic and pituitary system in normal foetuses. The drug is administered in the case of early diagnosis of CYP21A2 gene mutation in female foetuses [24].

7.4.2   Non-classical Congenital Adrenal Hyperplasia Due to 11-Beta-Hydroxylase Deficiency

Non-classical congenital hyperplasia due to 11-beta-hydroxylase deficiency results from CYP11B1 gene mutation. Absolute lack or deficiency of 11-beta-hydroxylase results in androgenisation along with cortisol deficiency and hypertension. Cortisol synthesis inhibition increases ACTH release. It results in adrenal hyperplasia and increased release of adrenal androgen, 11-deoxycorticosterone and 11-deoxycortisol.

Non-classical form is characteristic for its delayed onset of clinical symptoms. Baby girls are delivered with normal sexual organs, and only in their reproductive period, hirsutism and menstruation abnormalities (primary or secondary amenorrhea and oligomenorrhea) may appear [1]. Premature adrenarche and puberty are also very common as well as hypocalcaemia and hypertension.

In the diagnostic period, determination of 11-deoxycortisol and 11-deoxycorticosterone in serum, DHEAS, androstenedione and testosterone proves to be useful.

In the course of the therapy, hydrocortisone application until the puberty period and dexamethasone administration afterwards may provide good effects. If hypertension still persists, spironolactone or amiloride is recommended [25].

7.4.3 Addison's Disease

Addison's disease is a rare adrenal disorder characterised by low secretion of adrenocortical hormones. Female patients with Addison's disease may experience menstrual irregularity, but there is no sufficient data regarding the type of menstrual disturbance that is mostly observed in this rare disorder [1]. If Addison's disease is suspected, blood tests are carried out to measure the serum levels of sodium, potassium and cortisol. A low sodium, high potassium or low cortisol level may indicate Addison's disease.

7.5 Conclusions

Endocrine glands (pituitary, thyroid, adrenals) play a functional role in the endocrine regulation of a woman's menstrual cycle. In the simple diagram attached, we present the basic tests to be performed if secondary amenorrhoea is present and pituitary, thyroid and adrenal abnormalities are suspected (Fig. 7.1). As a result,

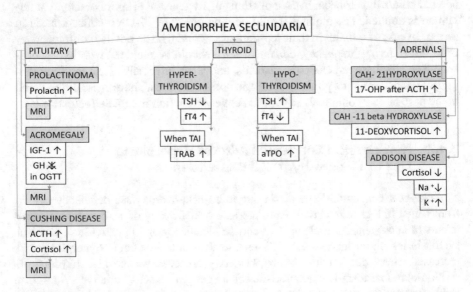

Fig. 7.1 Basic tests to be performed if secondary amenorrhoea is present and pituitary, thyroid and adrenal abnormalities are suspected

endocrine disorders are the triggers of onset of menstrual disturbance across the reproductive lifespan of women. Further studies are highly needed for better clarification of the underlying pathways of the association between endocrine disorders and menstrual cycle.

References

1. Saei Ghare Naz M, Rostami Dovom M, Ramezani Tehrani F. The menstrual disturbances in endocrine disorders: a narrative review. Int J Endocrinol Metab. 2020;18:e106694.
2. Kaltsas GA, Mukherjee JJ, Jenkins PJ, Satta MA, Islam N, Monson JP, et al. Menstrual irregularity in women with acromegaly. J Clin Endocrinol Metab. 1999;84:2731–5.
3. Katznelson L, Kleinberg D, Vance ML, Stavrou S, Pulaski KJ, Schoenfeld DA, et al. Hypogonadism in patients with acromegaly: data from the multi-centre acromegaly registry pilot study. Clin Endocrinol (Oxf). 2001;54:183–8.
4. Bolanowski M, Ruchała M, Zgliczyński W, Kos-Kudła B, Bałdys-Waligórska A, Zieliński G, et al. Acromegaly-a novel view of the patient. Polish proposals for diagnostic and therapeutic procedures in the light of recent reports. Endokrynol Pol. 2014;65:326–31.
5. Lado-Abeal J, Rodriguez-Arnao J, Newell-Price JD, Perry LA, Grossman AB, Besser GM, et al. Menstrual abnormalities in women with Cushing's disease are correlated with hypercortisolemia rather than raised circulating androgen levels. J Clin Endocrinol Metab. 1998;83:3083–8.
6. Aghajanova L, Stavreus-Evers A, Lindeberg M, Landgren BM, Sparre LS, Hovatta O. Thyroid-stimulating hormone receptor and thyroid hormone receptors are involved in human endometrial physiology. Fertil Steril. 2011;95:230–7.
7. Stavreus Evers A. Paracrine interactions of thyroid hormones and thyroid stimulation hormone in the female reproductive tract have an impact on female fertility. Front Endocrinol (Lausanne). 2012;3:50.
8. Catalano RD, Critchley HO, Heikinheimo O, Baird DT, Hapangama D, Sherwin JR, et al. Mifepristone induced progesterone withdrawal reveals novel regulatory pathways in human endometrium. Mol Hum Reprod. 2007;13:641–54.
9. Zhang SS, Carrillo AJ, Darling DS. Expression of multiple thyroid hormone receptor mRNAs in human oocytes, cumulus cells, and granulosa cells. Mol Hum Reprod. 1997;3:555–62.
10. Massimiani M, Lacconi V, La Civita F, Ticconi C, Rago R, Campagnolo L. Molecular signaling regulating endometrium-blastocyst crosstalk. Int J Mol Sci. 2019;21:23.
11. Koutras DA. Disturbances of menstruation in thyroid disease. Ann N Y Acad Sci. 1997;816:280–4.
12. Joshi JV, Bhandarkar SD, Chadha M, Balaiah D, Shah R. Menstrual irregularities and lactation failure may precede thyroid dysfunction or goitre. J Postgrad Med. 1993;39:137–41.
13. Unuane D, Velkeniers B. Impact of thyroid disease on fertility and assisted conception. Best Pract Res Clin Endocrinol Metab. 2020;34:101378.
14. Poppe K, Glinoer D, Van Steirteghem A, Tournaye H, Devroey P, Schiettecatte J, et al. Thyroid dysfunction and autoimmunity in infertile women. Thyroid. 2004;12:997–1001.
15. Koyyada A, Orsu P. Role of hypothyroidism and associated pathways in pregnancy and infertility: clinical insights. Tzu Chi Med J. 2020;32:312–7.
16. Poppe K. MANAGEMENT OF ENDOCRINE DISEASE: thyroid and female infertility: more questions than answers?! Eur J Endocrinol. 2021;184:R123–35.
17. Akande EO, Hockaday TD. Plasma oestrogen and luteinizing hormone concentrations in thyrotoxic menstrual disturbance. Proc R Soc Med. 1972;65:789–90.
18. Akande EO, Hockaday TDR. Plasma luteinizing hormone levels in women with thyrotoxicosis. J Endocrinol. 1972;53:173–4.

19. Akande EO. The effect of oestrogen on plasma levels of luteinizing hormone in euthyroid and thyrotoxic postmenopausal women. J Obstet Gynecol. 1974;81:795–803.
20. Pontikides N, Kaltsas T, Krassas GE. The hypothalamic-pituitary-gonadal axis in hyperthyroid female patients before and after treatment. J Endocrinol Investig. 1990;13(Suppl 2):203.
21. Zähringer S, Tomova A, von Werder K, Brabant G, Kumanov P, Schopohl J. The influence of hyperthyroidism on the hypothalamic-pituitary-gonadal axis. Exp Clin Endocrinol Diabetes. 2000;108:282–9.
22. Krassas GE, Markou KB. The impact of thyroid diseases starting from birth on reproductive function. Hormones (Athens). 2019;18:365–81.
23. Dumitrascu MC, Nenciu AE, Florica S, Nenciu CG, Petca A, Petca RC, et al. Hyperthyroidism management during pregnancy and lactation (Review). Exp Ther Med. 2021;22:960.
24. Livadas S, Bothou C. Management of the Female With Non-classical Congenital Adrenal Hyperplasia (NCCAH): A Patient-Oriented Approach. Front Endocrinol (Lausanne). 2019;10:366.
25. Kruse B, Riepe FG, Krone N, Bosinski HA, Kloehn S, Partsch CJ, et al. Congenital adrenal hyperplasia - how to improve the transition from adolescence to adult life. Exp Clin Endocrinol Diabetes. 2004;112:343–55.

Polycystic Ovarian Syndrome

8

Maria A. Christou, Gesthimani Mintziori,
Dimitrios G. Goulis, and Basil C. Tarlatzis

8.1 Introduction

Polycystic ovarian syndrome (PCOS) is a heterogeneous disorder and a prevalent cause of ovulatory and menstrual irregularity, infertility, hyperandrogenism, and metabolic dysfunction. It is one of the most common endocrine disorders in women of reproductive age, affecting 5–10% of women, depending upon the diagnostic criteria and the population studied [1]. Importantly, PCOS represents a significant financial burden to health care [2]. This chapter describes the different aspects of PCOS in premenopausal adult women, adolescents, and postmenopausal women.

8.2 Etiology

PCOS is a complex trait with multiple genetic and environmental intrauterine and extrauterine factors that interact to develop the disorder.

8.2.1 Genetic Factors

The genetic basis of PCOS was established by the increased prevalence of PCOS in first-degree female relatives of affected women, in female clustering and twin studies. Specifically, the largest twin study documented that genetic influences account for 70% of the variance in PCOS pathogenesis [3]. Additionally, the PCOS

M. A. Christou · G. Mintziori · D. G. Goulis · B. C. Tarlatzis (✉)
Units of Human Reproduction and Reproductive Endocrinology, 1st Department of Obstetrics and Gynecology, Medical School, Aristotle University of Thessaloniki, Thessaloniki, Greece
e-mail: gefsi@auth.gr; dgg@auth.gr

© International Society of Gynecological Endocrinology 2023
A. R. Genazzani et al. (eds.), *Amenorrhea*, ISGE Series,
https://doi.org/10.1007/978-3-031-22378-5_8

prevalence in mothers and sisters of PCOS women was 20–40%, considerably higher than that in the general population [4, 5].

Potentially responsible genes include those regulating gonadotropin secretion and action, ovarian folliculogenesis, insulin secretion and action, weight regulation, and androgen biosynthesis and action.

A recent overview systematically evaluated the evidence regarding PCOS genetics from candidate gene systematic reviews and genome-wide association studies (GWAS) [6]. The genetic loci with the most robust findings were in or near the genes *DENND1A, INS-VNTR,* and *INSR,* related to metabolism, and *THADA* and *FSHR,* implicated in the imbalance between gonadotropins and androgens. Other genes in susceptibility loci identified by GWAS were *LHCGR, HMGA2, RAB5B, SUOX, YAP,* and *ZNF217,* related to the gonadotropic axis, glucose and lipid metabolism, and cell cycle regulation [7]. Importantly, although the heritability of PCOS is approximately 70%, the proportion of heritability identified by GWAS is <10%. Thus, whole-exome sequencing is needed to screen the whole exome for rare variants with a large effect on the phenotype.

8.2.2 Environmental Factors

The most clearly defined environmental factor affecting PCOS development is diet and its association with obesity. Indeed, the genetic predisposition to PCOS seems to be exacerbated by weight gain and obesity. It has also been proposed that prenatal androgenization of the female fetus induced by genetic (e.g., variants determining androgen activity, variants determining androgen availability to target tissues) and/or environmental factors (e.g., exposure to chemical products, congenital adrenal hyperplasia, congenital adrenal virilizing tumors) may program differentiating target tissues toward the development of PCOS in later life [8].

Importantly, an association between PCOS development and exposure to endocrine-disrupting chemicals (EDCs) and advanced glycation end products (AGEs) has been described [9]. EDCs are exogenous substances, and AGEs are proinflammatory molecules derived from nonenzymatic glycation and oxidation of proteins and lipids or are absorbed from exogenous sources. Dietary and environmental exposure to EDCs and AGEs through different life cycle stages may alter the reproductive system's function and PCOS development. They may also lead to metabolic disturbance (e.g., obesity, insulin resistance, hyperinsulinemia) that can exacerbate the PCOS phenotype and contribute to PCOS health risks such as type 2 diabetes mellitus (T2DM) and cardiovascular disease.

8.3 Pathophysiology

The proposed pathophysiology of PCOS is an interaction between impaired gonadotropin secretion and action, dysfunction in ovarian folliculogenesis, ovarian and adrenal hyperandrogenism, and insulin resistance accompanied by hyperinsulinemia [6].

Altered luteinizing hormone (LH) action appears to be involved in PCOS pathophysiology. Specifically, women with PCOS often have higher serum LH concentrations [10] and increased LH pulse frequency and amplitude than matched controls [11]. Additionally, the LH receptor is overexpressed in thecal and granulosa cells from polycystic ovaries [12]. However, serum LH tends to be lower in obese women with PCOS compared with lean counterparts [13].

Indeed, the progesterone peak does not occur through a luteal phase of the menstrual cycle in PCOS women, and the frequency and amplitude of gonadotropin-releasing hormone (GnRH) pulses are increased, leading to increased LH and subsequently increased androgen synthesis and secretion in the ovaries. Although the ovaries are the main source of androgens in PCOS, increased adrenal androgens [mainly dehydroepiandrosterone (DHEA) and dehydroepiandrosterone sulfate (DHEAS)] are present in 20–30% of women with PCOS [14].

The increase in follicular androgens impairs follicular development to dominant follicles and reduces the inhibition of GnRH pulse frequency by progesterone [15]. Although follicle-stimulating hormone (FSH) levels are generally normal, follicles seem to be resistant to FSH, which might be in part due to increased anti-mullerian hormone (AMH) [16]. In this way, high AMH levels inhibit FSH-dependent follicular maturation and selection of dominant follicles and inhibit FSH-induced aromatase expression, leading to hyperandrogenism.

Insulin resistance and hyperinsulinemia are frequent findings in PCOS [17], with the etiology remaining unclear. However, a post-binding defect in receptor signaling affecting glucose transporter-4 (GLUT-4) expression and thus insulin target tissues, such as adipose tissue, muscle, and possibly the ovary, has been described [18]. Specifically, a defect in serine phosphorylation of the insulin receptor that results in decreased activation of the receptor has been identified in 50% of women with PCOS [19].

Hyperinsulinemia stimulates the secretion of androgens from theca cells [20] and inhibits hepatic sex hormone-binding globulin (SHBG) production [21], increasing free androgens.

8.4 Diagnostic Criteria and Different Phenotypes

8.4.1 Diagnostic Criteria

Most experts use the Rotterdam criteria to diagnose PCOS because they are the most inclusive [22, 23]. They were developed at a 2003 consensus meeting held in Rotterdam [European Society of Human Reproduction and Embryology (ESHRE) and American Society for Reproductive Medicine (ASRM) consensus workshop group]. Specifically, two of the following three criteria are required to make the diagnosis:

- Oligo- and/or anovulation
- Clinical and/or biochemical hyperandrogenism
- Polycystic ovarian-like morphology (PCOM) by ultrasound

Table 8.1 PCOS diagnostic criteria and phenotypes in adult women

	Phenotypes			
	A	B	C	D
Features				
Hyperandrogenism	✓	✓	✓	
Ovulatory dysfunction	✓	✓		✓
PCOM	✓		✓	✓
Diagnostic criteria				
NIH 1990	✓	✓		
AE-PCOS 2006	✓	✓	✓	
ASRM/ESHRE 2003	✓	✓	✓	✓

Abbreviations: *AE-PCOS* Androgen Excess and PCOS Society, *ASRM* American Society for Reproductive Medicine, *ESHRE* European Society of Human Reproduction and Embryology, *NIH* National Institutes of Health, *PCOM* polycystic ovarian-like morphology, *PCOS* polycystic ovarian syndrome
All diagnostic criteria require exclusion of other conditions that may mimic PCOS clinical picture

PCOS diagnosis is confirmed only when other conditions that mimic PCOS are excluded.

These criteria, with minor adjustments, have been reaffirmed by a recent international evidence-based guideline for the assessment and management of PCOS [24]. Other proposed criteria include the 1990 National Institutes of Health (NIH) criteria and the criteria proposed in 2006 from the Androgen Excess and PCOS (AEPCOS) Society (AE-PCOS criteria) (Table 8.1) [25, 26].

PCOS prevalence varies according to the diagnostic criteria used to define the disorder. Specifically, in a 2016 meta-analysis of 24 population studies performed in Europe, Australia, Asia, and the United States, PCOS rates (95% confidence intervals, CI) according to the NIH criteria, the Rotterdam criteria, and the AE-PCOS criteria were 6% (5–8%, 18 trials), 10% (8–13%, 15 trials), and 10% (7–13%, 10 trials), respectively, in unselected reproductive-aged women [1].

Importantly, the prevalence of PCOS is increased in obesity, insulin resistance, diabetes mellitus (type 1, type 2, or gestational), oligoovulatory infertility, premature adrenarche, family history of PCOS in first-degree relatives, and certain ethnic groups (e.g., Indigenous Australians) [27].

8.4.2 Phenotypes

The Rotterdam criteria yield four different PCOS phenotypes:

- Phenotype A: includes hyperandrogenism (biochemical and/or clinical), ovulatory dysfunction, and PCOM
- Phenotype B: includes hyperandrogenism (biochemical and/or clinical) and ovulatory dysfunction

- Phenotype C: includes hyperandrogenism (biochemical and/or clinical) and PCOM
- Phenotype D: includes ovulatory dysfunction and PCOM

Notably, the NIH criteria include only phenotypes A and B; the AE-PCOS criteria phenotypes A, B, and C; and the Rotterdam criteria all phenotypes (Table 8.1). Epidemiological studies in unselected populations have shown that the prevalence of phenotypes A and B was 40–45%, ~35% for phenotype C, and ~20% for phenotype D [28].

8.5   Evaluation

The main features of PCOS include androgen excess (biochemically and/or clinically), menstrual irregularity, and/or PCOM. There are several proposed diagnostic criteria for PCOS, all of which require that other causes of menstrual irregularity and hyperandrogenism should be excluded.

8.5.1   Menstrual Irregularity

The menstrual irregularity in PCOS is caused by infrequent or absent ovulation. It usually has a peripubertal onset, and affected women may have a normal or slightly delayed menarche followed by irregular cycles. Other women may have regular cycles at first and subsequently develop menstrual irregularity in association with weight gain. PCOS women often experience more regular cycles after the age of 40 years. Women who develop menstrual irregularity at a later age (e.g., >30 years) are less likely to have PCOS.

Oligoovulation or anovulation in PCOS leads to a decrease in progesterone secretion. Thus, women with PCOS may have constant mitogenic stimulation of the endometrium due to an increase in estrogen and absence of endometrium differentiation due to a decrease in progesterone. This fact leads to abnormal intermittent uterine bleeding [29].

Thus, menstrual irregularity in PCOS women could be:

- Amenorrhea
  - Primary amenorrhea: lack of menarche by 15 years of age (or by 15 years' bone age if puberty onset was early) or >3 years post-thelarche (breast development)
  - Secondary amenorrhea: >90 days without a menstrual period in previously menstruating girls (>1 year post-menarche)
- Oligomenorrhea
  - <1 year post-menarche: normal as part of the pubertal transition
  - 1–3 years post-menarche: average cycle length >45 days
  - 3 years post-menarche–perimenopause: average cycle length >35 days or <8 menstrual periods per year

- Dysfunctional uterine bleeding
  - Frequent bleeding: bleeding <21 days (<19 days in <1 year post-menarche)
  - Prolonged bleeding: bleeding lasting >7 days in adolescents or >8 days in adults
  - Heavy bleeding: soaking pads or tampons sufficiently to interfere with the physical, social, emotional, or material quality of life

8.5.2 Hyperandrogenism

Hyperandrogenism may include clinical signs and/or elevated serum androgen concentrations. Most PCOS women have both clinical and biochemical evidence of hyperandrogenism.

8.5.2.1 Clinical Hyperandrogenism

Hyperandrogenism in PCOS is manifested clinically by hirsutism, acne, and/or balding with potential negative psychosocial impact. Hirsutism is present in about 70% of women with PCOS, whereas acne and balding are not commonly present.

The majority of hirsutism is due to androgen excess ($\geq$80%) [30]. However, hirsutism may occur without elevated androgen concentrations (idiopathic hirsutism). Hirsutism should be distinguished from hypertrichosis distributed in a non-sexual pattern and is not caused by androgen excess.

Hirsutism is defined as excess terminal (>0.5 cm length, pigmented) body hair in a male pattern. The modified Ferriman-Gallwey (mFG) visual scale is preferred to evaluate hirsutism in the most androgen-sensitive areas [31]. Nine body areas (upper lip, chin, chest, arm, upper abdomen, lower abdomen, upper back, lower back, thighs) are scored from 1 (minimal terminal hairs) to 4 (equivalent to a hairy man). If no terminal hairs are observed, then the score 0 is given. A mFG score $\geq$4–6 indicates hirsutism, acknowledging that self-treatment is common and can limit clinical assessment. Importantly, there is substantial racial variability in hirsutism, defined as a mFG score of $\geq$9–10 in Mediterranean populations, $\geq$8 in the US population, and $\geq$2–3 in Asian populations [32].

Acne as an isolated sign might not be considered a hyperandrogenic sign. However, hyperandrogenism should be considered when it is severe or combined with hirsutism or menstrual irregularity [33]. Acne occurs in adolescence and may persist into adulthood. It presents most commonly on the face, neck, chest, shoulders, and back. Balding may be either a male pattern (affecting the fronto-temporo-occipital scalp) or a female pattern (affecting the crown) [34]. The Ludwig visual scale is preferred for assessing the degree and distribution of balding, whereas there are no universally accepted visual scales for evaluating acne.

8.5.2.2 Biochemical Hyperandrogenism

In women with hyperandrogenic signs, calculated free testosterone, free androgen index (FAI), or calculated bioavailable testosterone should be measured to assess biochemical hyperandrogenism. Calculations of free testosterone and bioavailable testosterone can be carried out using the formula available on the website of the International Society for the Study of the Aging Male (ISSAM) (http://www.issam.ch/freetesto.htm) from total testosterone, SHBG, and albumin values measured in the same sample for each subject. FAI can be calculated according to the following equation: FAI = [total testosterone (nmol/L)/SHBG (nmol/L)] × 100%. Serum total or free testosterone is best assessed by high-quality assays, such as liquid chromatography-tandem mass spectroscopy (LC-MS) and extraction/chromatography immunoassays. The upper limit of normal for serum testosterone in women is 45–60 ng/dL (1.6–2.1 nmol/L) measured by LC-MS.

DHEAS and androstenedione provide limited additional information in PCOS diagnosis and could be measured if total or free testosterone is not elevated. DHEAS is also suggested to be measured in severe hyperandrogenism because it can be very high in adrenocortical tumors. Additionally, in the case of biochemical hyperandrogenism, a morning serum 17-hydroxyprogesterone [17(OH)P] should be measured to rule out non-classic congenital adrenal hyperplasia (NCCAH) due to 21-hydroxylase deficiency. This measurement should be done in the early follicular phase for women with spontaneous menstrual cycles, whereas it should be done on a random day for those without cycles.

Reliable assessment of biochemical hyperandrogenism is not possible in women on hormonal contraception due to effects on SHBG and gonadotropin-dependent androgen production. Thus, drug withdrawal is recommended for at least 3 months before measurement.

8.5.3 PCOM

Transvaginal, rather than transabdominal, ultrasound should be performed to determine the presence of PCOM if sexually active. The main ovarian finding in PCOS is multiple, small, preantral, and antral follicles in a peripheral location with an increased volume of the stroma. Importantly, follicle number and size are relevant to an ultrasound diagnosis. The Rotterdam ultrasound criteria include ≥12 follicles in each ovary (2–9 mm in diameter) and/or increased ovarian volume (>10 mL), ensuring that no corpora lutea, cysts, or dominant follicles are present. Follicle number and ovarian volume decrease with age in women with or without PCOS. The International PCOS Network has proposed revised criteria for PCOS, confirming an ovarian volume >10 mL and suggesting an increase in follicle number ≥20 follicles per ovary, using transducers with a frequency bandwidth that includes 8 MHz [24]. In the case of using older transvaginal technology or performing transabdominal ultrasound, an ovarian volume >10 mL is needed, given the difficulty of reliably assessing follicle number with this approach.

8.5.4   Other Biochemical Characteristics

Most commonly, women with PCOS have an increase in LH concentrations and LH pulse frequency and amplitude [13]. The likelihood of finding increased serum LH depends upon the sample timing relative to the last menstrual period, the ovarian activity, the use of combined oral contraceptives (COCs), and the body mass index (BMI). Therefore, the absence of increased serum LH does not exclude PCOS diagnosis.

Serum FSH levels may be normal or low in PCOS women. In the past, many clinicians used an elevated LH/FSH ratio of ≥ 2 for PCOS diagnosis. However, its use may be misleading. Specifically, if there has been recent ovulation, LH will be suppressed, and the ratio will be ≤ 2.

In women with intermenstrual intervals >35 days, serum progesterone (additionally to ultrasound) can be measured to assess whether ovulation has occurred. In normally cycling women, this is done on day 21 of a cycle. However, in women with long intermenstrual intervals, progesterone is measured 7–10 days before the next menses is expected. Importantly, ovulatory dysfunction can still occur with regular cycles, and if ovulation needs to be confirmed, serum progesterone can be measured.

Serum AMH is produced by small (<8 mm) preantral and early antral follicles, reflecting the number of primordial follicles. As already mentioned, follicular development is abnormal in PCOS. Growth of antral follicles tends to be arrested at 5–8 mm in diameter, much smaller than a mature follicle. In one study, serum AMH concentrations were two- to threefold higher in PCOS women compared with controls [35], and also a meta-analysis suggested that a serum AMH >4.7 ng/mL had a 79% specificity and an 83% sensitivity to diagnose PCOS [36]. Generally, serum AMH concentrations are in the upper range of normal or markedly elevated in women with PCOS [37]. However, AMH assays are limited by the absence of an international standard, and an increased AMH should not be considered as a criterion for PCOS diagnosis.

8.6   Differential Diagnosis

Oligomenorrhea can also be seen in hypothyroidism, hyperthyroidism, hyperprolactinemia, and ovarian insufficiency. However, these disorders are distinguished by their clinical characteristics (hyperandrogenic signs are not common) and biochemical testing. Therefore, additional testing should be performed in any woman with oligomenorrhea, including thyroid-stimulating hormone (TSH), prolactin, and FSH. Hypogonadotropic hypogonadism, due to low body fat or intensive exercise, should also be excluded clinically and biochemically (LH and FSH levels). A serum or urine pregnancy test should be performed to rule out pregnancy.

The clinical characteristics of NCCAH can be similar to PCOS (mild hyperandrogenism, oligomenorrhea, PCOM). Affected women may also present with premature pubarche. NCCAH should be ruled out because there are risks that offspring could be affected with the more severe classic 21-hydroxylase deficiency. A morning value of 17(OH)P >200 ng/dL (6 nmol/L) in the early follicular phase strongly suggests the diagnosis, which may be confirmed by a high-dose (250 µg) adrenocorticotropic hormone (ACTH) stimulation test with most patients with the diagnosis having 17(OH)P >1500 ng/dL (43 nmol/L).

Additionally, Cushing syndrome may be associated with hyperandrogenic anovulation [38]. Acromegaly is also associated with PCOS [39]. Specifically, the elevated levels of insulin-like growth factor-1 (IGF-1) in acromegaly can cause PCOS by increasing the activity of multiple steroidogenic enzymes in the ovaries and adrenals.

For women with clinical signs of severe hyperandrogenism (e.g., severe hirsutism, frontal balding, severe acne, clitoromegaly, increased muscle mass, deepening of the voice) of recent onset that is rapidly progressive, serum total testosterone and DHEAS should be measured. These women (usually postmenopausal) probably have an androgen-secreting tumor (ovarian or adrenal) or ovarian hyperthecosis. In these cases, serum total testosterone concentrations are almost always >150 ng/dL (5.2 nmol/L) [40] and, in the case of adrenal tumors, serum DHEAS concentrations are >800 µg/dL (21.6 µmol/L). Notably, anabolic-androgenic steroid use may present with features similar to those of virilizing tumors.

Approximately 8% of hyperandrogenic patients have no identifiable ovarian or adrenal source of increased androgens, and the diagnosis of idiopathic hyperandrogenism is given.

8.7 Health Risks

8.7.1 Metabolic Health Risks

8.7.1.1 Weight Gain and Obesity

There is an increased weight gain and obesity prevalence in PCOS, increasing the severity of the condition [41]. In one study in Spain, the prevalence of obesity was 51% in women with PCOS and 18% in the group of controls [42]. In another study from the United States, 60% of women with PCOS were obese [43], twice the rate seen in the general population [44]. However, obesity prevalence in PCOS varies widely with the population studied [45], suggesting that environmental factors play a significant role in determining obesity in PCOS.

8.7.1.2 Impaired Glucose Tolerance (IGT): Type 2 Diabetes Mellitus (T2DM)

Regardless of age, the risk of IGT and T2DM is significantly increased in PCOS women, especially those with a first-degree relative with T2DM, with risk independent of, yet exacerbated by, obesity [46, 47]. Specifically, in a study of 122 obese women with PCOS, 45% had IGT and 10% had T2DM by age 40 years [46]. The latter women had a 2.6-fold higher prevalence of first-degree relatives with T2DM. Importantly, the annual conversion rate from normal glucose tolerance to IGT was 16% in another study of 71 women with PCOS [48].

8.7.1.3　Dyslipidemia

Most studies of women with PCOS have shown low high-density lipoprotein cholesterol (HDL-c), high low-density lipoprotein cholesterol (LDL-c), and high tri-
glyceride concentrations [49]. For example, in a study of 398 women with PCOS,
the prevalence of abnormal lipids was quite high; 35% had total cholesterol
≥200 mg/dL, 31% had LDL-c ≥130 mg/dL, 15% had HDL-c <35 mg/dL, and 16%
had triglycerides >200 mg/dL [50].

8.7.1.4　Insulin Resistance

Most women with PCOS are insulin resistant and hyperinsulinemic compared with
controls, independent of obesity [51, 52]. However, it is not possible to determine
the extent to which PCOS contributes to insulin resistance independent of obesity,
and there is currently no validated test for measuring insulin resistance in a clinical
setting [53]. The clinical manifestations of insulin resistance include acanthosis
nigricans, metabolic syndrome, nonalcoholic fatty liver disease, and sleep apnea.

8.7.1.5　Metabolic Syndrome

In the latest report (1999–2000) of the National Health and Nutrition Examination
Survey (NHANES), the prevalence of the metabolic syndrome (as defined by the
National Cholesterol Education Program/Adult Treatment Panel III criteria) in normal women aged 20–39 years was 18–19% [54]. Using the same diagnostic criteria,
the prevalence of the metabolic syndrome is much higher (43%) in PCOS
women [55].

Importantly, glycemic status, BMI, waist circumference, fasting lipids, and blood
pressure should be assessed at initial diagnosis in all women with PCOS. Glycemic
status includes fasting plasma glucose and a 75 g oral glucose tolerance test (OGTT)
or hemoglobin A1c. The OGTT is recommended in high-risk women (e.g., BMI
>25 kg/m^2, history of impaired fasting glucose, IGT or gestational diabetes, family
history of T2DM, hypertension, or high-risk ethnicity group). PCOS women with
normal glucose tolerance should be rescreened every 1–3 years or more frequently
if additional risk factors are identified, whereas those with impaired glucose tolerance should be screened annually for the development of T2DM.

Monitoring for weight changes and excess weight should be performed in every
visit or at least every 6–12 months. Additionally, overweight and obese PCOS
women, irrespective of age, should have a fasting lipid profile measurement. The
frequency of measurement should be based on the presence of hyperlipidemia and
total cardiovascular risk. Blood pressure should also be measured annually or more
frequently based on total cardiovascular risk.

8.7.1.6　Nonalcoholic Fatty Liver Disease (NAFLD)

NAFLD prevalence, including nonalcoholic steatohepatitis (NASH), may be
increased in women with PCOS [56, 57]. Notably, metformin and thiazolidinediones have been considered a possible therapy for women with PCOS who also have
NASH. However, routine screening for NAFLD in women with PCOS is not
suggested.

8.7.1.7 Sleep Apnea

It has been shown that sleep apnea is associated with PCOS, with the severity of sleep apnea correlating with the number of features of the metabolic syndrome present [58]. Specifically, obstructive sleep apnea and excessive daytime sleepiness were significantly more common in PCOS women compared with controls, odds ratio (OR) 30.6 (95% CI 7.2–139.4) and OR 9.0 (95% CI 4.0–22.1), respectively [59]. It was also shown that obstructive sleep apnea is an important determinant of insulin resistance, glucose intolerance, and T2DM in PCOS women [60]. Importantly, PCOS women should be asked about signs and symptoms of sleep apnea (snoring, waking unrefreshed from sleep, excessive daytime sleepiness, morning headaches) using a simple screening questionnaire, preferably the Berlin tool. If the diagnosis is suspected, the patient should be referred to a sleep medicine clinician.

8.7.2 Cardiovascular Health Risks

Women with PCOS present metabolic risk factors for premature coronary heart disease, such as obesity, insulin resistance, IGT, T2DM, dyslipidemia, hypertension, and/or metabolic syndrome in general [61, 62]. However, the increased frequency of cardiovascular events in women with PCOS is not well established [63]. Additionally, a meta-analysis has shown a twofold risk of arterial disease for women with PCOS compared to women without PCOS after BMI adjustment, suggesting that the increased risk of cardiovascular events in PCOS is not completely related to a higher BMI [64]. Nevertheless, all women with PCOS should be assessed for cardiovascular risk factors and total cardiovascular risk. Women should be considered at increased cardiovascular disease risk in the presence of related risk factors, such as obesity, dyslipidemia, hypertension, IGT, smoking, and lack of physical activity.

8.7.3 Gynecological Health Risks

8.7.3.1 Endometrial Cancer

In PCOS, chronic stimulation of the endometrium by estrogen, in the presence of chronically low progesterone secretion associated with anovulation, may increase the risk of endometrial hyperplasia and cancer, even before menopause [65]. Women with PCOS may also have other risk factors for endometrial cancer, including obesity, chronic hyperinsulinemia, and increased serum IGF-1 concentrations [66].

A meta-analysis of five studies including 138 women with PCOS and 5593 controls without PCOS reported an increased risk of endometrial cancer among women with PCOS (OR 2.79, 95% CI 1.31–5.95) [67]. It has also been suggested that in oligoovulatory women with PCOS, an endometrial thickness <7 mm on transvaginal ultrasound was not associated with histologic evidence of endometrial hyperplasia [68].

However, it is not suggested to use ultrasound routinely in premenopausal women with PCOS to screen for the presence of endometrial hyperplasia or cancer. An investigation by transvaginal ultrasound and/or endometrial biopsy is recommended with persistent thickened endometrium and/or relevant risk factors, including prolonged amenorrhea, abnormal vaginal bleeding, or excess weight. Prevention of endometrial hyperplasia could include COCs or progestin therapy in women with a cycle length >90 days.

8.7.3.2 Pregnancy Complications

The risk of pregnancy complications is increased in women with PCOS. The spontaneous abortion rate is 20–40% higher in PCOS women than in the general population [69]. Additionally, in a meta-analysis of 27 studies involving 4982 women with PCOS, the ORs (95% CI) of developing gestational diabetes, pregnancy-induced hypertension, preeclampsia, and preterm birth were 3.43 (2.49–4.74), 3.43 (2.49–4.74), 2.17 (1.91–2.46), and 1.93 (1.45–2.57), respectively, compared with the general population [70]. Furthermore, their babies had a higher risk of admission to the neonatal intensive care unit (OR 2.32, 95% CI 1.40–3.85). It has been suggested that the low-grade, chronic inflammation seen in PCOS women, as evidenced by high serum C-reactive protein concentrations, worsens during pregnancy and may be associated with an increased risk of pregnancy complications [71].

Importantly, a 75gr OGTT should be offered to all women with PCOS preconception, given the high risk of hyperglycemia and related comorbidities in pregnancy. If the OGTT is not performed preconception, then it should be offered at <20 weeks' gestation, and also all women with PCOS should perform the test at 24–28 weeks' gestation.

8.7.3.3 Infertility

PCOS is one of the most common cause of infertility with anovulation being the main pathophysiological mechanism. Women are encouraged to consider conceiving before 35 years to allow time for fertility interventions if needed.

8.7.4 Psychosocial Health Risks

There is a high prevalence of moderate-to-severe mood disorders (depression and anxiety) in women with PCOS and a likely increased prevalence in adolescents. Interestingly, it is suggested that women with PCOS are more likely to have mood disorders when compared with women without PCOS that are not always explained by features of PCOS such as obesity or hyperandrogenic signs [72]. All women with PCOS should be screened for mood disorders at the time of diagnosis [73], and where necessary, they should be referred for appropriate support. Women with PCOS are also at risk for eating disorders, particularly binge eating and bulimia nervosa [74], psychosexual dysfunction, negative body image concern, and diminished quality of life.

8.8   Treatment

The approach to management depends on the woman's life stage, medical history, concerns, and preferences. COCs, metformin, and other pharmacological treatments are generally off-label in PCOS. However, their use is evidence based and is allowed in many countries. Tables 8.2 and 8.3 describe the advantages and disadvantages of the treatment options in PCOS for non-fertility and fertility indications, respectively. The goals of therapy are the following:

- Management of metabolic abnormalities
- Management of menstrual irregularity
- Prevention of endometrial hyperplasia and cancer
- Contraception for those not pursuing pregnancy
- Management of hyperandrogenic characteristics
- Ovulation induction for those pursuing pregnancy

Table 8.2 Treatment for non-fertility indications in women with PCOS

Line	Agent	Advantages	Disadvantages
First	Weight loss (if overweight/obese)	• Overall health benefits • Metabolic, reproductive, and psychological benefits	• Time-consuming process • Difficulty to avoid weight regain in the long term
First	COCs	• Management of menstrual irregularity • Prevention of endometrial hyperplasia • Contraception • Management of hyperandrogenemia	• Off-label use • Venous thrombosis • Arterial thrombosis (e.g., MI, ischemic stroke) • Impaired lipid metabolism • Many absolute and relative contraindications
First	Progestin-only preparations	• Alternative option in case of contraindications or intolerance to COCs • Third- and fourth-generation progestins cause fewer metabolic adverse effects • Fourth-generation progestins are antiandrogenic • Few absolute contraindications (e.g., current breast cancer, unexplained vaginal bleeding, intrauterine infection)	• Very few data in women with PCOS • Less effective compared to COCs

(continued)

Table 8.2 (continued)

Line	Agent	Advantages	Disadvantages
Second	COCs + metformin	• Considered in high-risk metabolic groups or for management of metabolic features	
Second	COCs + antiandrogen	• Considered for hyperandrogenic signs when ≥6 months of COCs with cosmetic therapy has failed	• Antiandrogens must be used with contraception to prevent male fetal virilization
Second	Metformin	• Improves BMI, menstrual cyclicity, androgen levels, and metabolic features	• Off-label use • Dose-dependent gastrointestinal disorders • Decreased vitamin B_{12} • More effective agents for non-fertility indications are available

Abbreviations: *BMI* body mass index, *COCs* combined oral contraceptives, *MI* myocardial infarction, *PCOS* polycystic ovarian syndrome

Table 8.3 Treatment for fertility in women with PCOS

Line	Agent	Advantages	Disadvantages
First	Weight loss	• Low cost • Overall health, metabolic, reproductive, and psychological benefits	• Time-consuming process • Difficulty to avoid weight regain in the long term
First	Letrozole	• Oral • Low cost • Compared to clomiphene citrate – Higher ovulation, pregnancy, and live birth rates – Lower time to pregnancy – Lower multiple pregnancy risk	• Off-label use
First	Clomiphene citrate	• Oral • Low cost • Preferred in obese women compared to metformin	• Compared with letrozole – Lower ovulation, pregnancy, and live birth rates – Higher time to pregnancy – Higher multiple pregnancy risk

Table 8.3 (continued)

Line	Agent	Advantages	Disadvantages
First	Clomiphene citrate + metformin	• Improve ovulation, pregnancy, live birth rates, and time to pregnancy in obese women • Decrease time to pregnancy in clomiphene citrate-resistant women	
First	Metformin	• Oral • Low cost • Safe • Improves ovulation, pregnancy, and live birth rates	• Off-label use • Dose-dependent gastrointestinal disorders • Decreased vitamin B_{12} • More effective ovulation induction agents are available
Second	Gonadotropins	• Comparable pregnancy and live birth rates to ovarian drilling	• Daily injections • High cost • Multiple pregnancy risk • OHSS risk • Frequent medical monitoring
Second	Ovarian drilling	• Performed once • Minimally invasive • Normalizes ultrasonographic findings • Restores ovulatory cycles for many years • Compared to gonadotropins: – Comparable pregnancy and live birth rates – Lower risk of multiple pregnancies or OHSS • Improves response to IVF	• High cost • Surgical risk • Postoperative adhesions • Diminished ovarian reserve
Third	ART	• IVF – Decreased multiple pregnancy rate by SET and/or freeze-all – Similar pregnancy rate compared to women without PCOS	• Very high cost • Invasive procedure • OHSS risk

Abbreviations: *ART* assisted reproduction technology, *IVF* in vitro fertilization, *OHSS* ovarian hyperstimulation syndrome, *PCOS* polycystic ovarian syndrome, *SET* single-embryo transfer

8.8.1 Metabolic Abnormalities

A healthy lifestyle and prevention of weight gain are important for all women with PCOS from adolescence to menopause. Lifestyle interventions (diet, physical activity, and/or behavioral counseling) are suggested for weight reduction as the first step for overweight and obese women with PCOS [75], followed by pharmacotherapy [76] and, when necessary, bariatric surgery [77]. Modest weight loss of 5–10% within 6 months in those PCOS women with excess weight is recommended.

General healthy eating principles should be followed for all women with PCOS across the life course, as per general population recommendations. Calorie-restricted diets (energy deficit of 30% or 500–750 kcal/day) are suggested for women with PCOS and excess weight. However, there is no good evidence that one type of diet is superior to another [78]. Physical activity (planned or unplanned in the context of daily, family, and community activities) should be advised for prevention of weight gain, weight loss, prevention of weight regain, and greater health benefits.

Importantly, in addition to lifestyle, metformin should be considered in over-weight or obese women with PCOS to manage weight and metabolic outcomes. Metformin may offer greater benefit in high-risk metabolic groups such as IGT, diabetes, or high-risk ethnic groups. In addition to metformin, thiazolidinediones can reduce insulin levels in women with PCOS [79, 80]. However, because of limited clinical data, potential weight gain, and a possible association with cardiovascular adverse events, the use of thiazolidinediones is not recommended in women with PCOS who do not have diabetes. Other anti-obesity medications (e.g., glucagon-like peptide-1 analogs, naltrexone/bupropion combination) could be considered for managing obesity in women with PCOS, as per general population recommendations considering cost, contraindications, and side effects.

8.8.2 Menstrual Irregularity: Endometrial Protection

When a menstrual irregularity is presented in overweight or obese women with PCOS, 5–10% weight loss could help restore normal ovulatory cycles [81, 82].

COCs are suggested as the first-line therapy for menstrual irregularity and endometrial protection [24]. The approach to COCs use is the same as in women without PCOS. They provide several benefits in women with PCOS:

- Exposure to progestin, which antagonizes the endometrial proliferative effect of estrogen
- Contraception in those not pursuing pregnancy, as women with oligomenorrhea ovulate intermittently and an unwanted pregnancy may occur
- Cutaneous benefits for hyperandrogenic signs

No specific preparation is superior in PCOS, with all agents increasing SHBG and improving clinical outcomes. When prescribing COCs, the lowest effective estrogen dose (such as 20–30 µg ethinyloestradiol or equivalent) is preferred balancing efficacy, metabolic risk profile, side effects, cost, and availability, and 35 µg ethinyloestradiol is not recommended as a first-line treatment.

COCs increase the risk of venous thromboembolism (VTE) related to both the dose of estrogen and the type of progestin. VTE incidence is 5–10 events per 10,000 woman-years in the general population and 8–10 events per 10,000 woman-years in COCs users, lower than the pregnancy-related VTE incidence (1.2 events every 1,000 deliveries) [83]. However, it is unclear if COCs constitute an independent risk factor for VTE, given that PCOS is a prothrombotic state itself. All PCOS women should be evaluated for cardiometabolic risk factors at baseline before initiating a COC. Age, smoking, obesity, glucose intolerance or diabetes, hypertension, dyslipidemia, thrombophilia, and family history of VTE should be recorded and guide treatment options.

Arterial thrombotic events related to COCs use occur much less frequently. Overall arterial thrombosis risk (myocardial infarction or ischemic stroke) in COCs users was 1.6-fold increased [84]. Importantly, current data do not suggest adverse effects of COCs on glucose metabolism, whereas COCs may increase serum levels of triglycerides, LDL-c, and HDL-c mainly due to their effects on the liver [83].

For those women with PCOS who choose not to or cannot take COCs, alternative treatments for endometrial protection are intermittent or continuous progestin use or a progestin-releasing intrauterine device. Importantly, progestin alone will not reduce hyperandrogenic signs, nor will it provide contraception.

Metformin is another alternative as it restores menstrual cyclicity in 30–50% of women with PCOS [85]. However, it is considered a second-line therapy [24]. The combination of COCs and metformin should be considered for high-risk metabolic groups or management of metabolic features when COCs and lifestyle changes do not achieve the desired goals.

8.8.3 Hyperandrogenism

The general treatment of skin problems focuses on reducing androgen production, decreasing the fraction of free testosterone, and limiting androgen bioactivity at the target tissues.

A COC combined with cosmetic therapy (e.g., shaving, waxing, depilatories, electrolysis, or laser treatment in the case of hirsutism) is suggested as a first-line pharmacologic therapy in most women with hyperandrogenic signs, as the former decreases ovarian androgen production, suppressing LH secretion and increasing SHBG [30]. An antiandrogen is then added after 6 months if the cosmetic response is suboptimal. Importantly, pregnancy should be ruled out before starting COCs or antiandrogens. Typically, cyproterone acetate is a fourth-generation progestin with the greatest antiandrogen activity of all progestins, which, due to significant VTE risk, is used to treat moderate-to-severe hyperandrogenic signs. Additionally, spironolactone can be added 50–100 mg twice daily. Other antiandrogens include finasteride (inhibits 5-alpha-reductase type 2, which converts testosterone to dihydrotestosterone), cyproterone acetate, and flutamide.

COCs and an antiandrogen may be started simultaneously, particularly in the case of severe cutaneous manifestations. However, the antiandrogen is started usually after the completion of at least 1 month of taking COCs. When COCs are contraindicated or poorly tolerated, an antiandrogen may be used alone in women with hirsutism. However, an alternative form of contraception is needed because an antiandrogen could prevent the development of normal external genitalia in a male fetus in the case of pregnancy. Importantly, an antiandrogen alone does not regularize menstrual cycles.

8.8.4 Ovulation Induction and Fertility

The "Consensus on Infertility Treatment Related to PCOS," held in Thessaloniki in 2007 [86] and, more recently, the "International Evidence-Based Guideline for the Assessment and Management of PCOS" [24] addressed all fertility treatment options for PCOS women. The treatment choice should result from a joint decision between the infertile couple and the medical team based on a woman's special characteristics and the couple's wishes.

Several factors that affect fertility (e.g., glycemic status, blood pressure, weight, smoking, alcohol) should be assessed and optimized in women with PCOS before initiating ovulation induction. Additionally, pregnancy needs to be excluded, as well as fallopian tube patency should be assessed.

8.8.4.1 Weight Loss

Lifestyle changes to induce weight loss are considered the first-line therapy for infertility in obese women with PCOS being implemented before ovulation induction. Importantly, obesity is an independent risk factor for anovulation, failed or delayed response to treatment, first-trimester miscarriages, and third-trimester complications. Thus, a modest weight loss (5–10%) in overweight or obese women is suggested to restore fertility.

Although weight loss is encouraged in obese women with PCOS and anovulatory infertility, women are referred to a fertility specialist if they cannot conceive after lifestyle changes for 12 months and 6 months if aged <35 years and >35 years, respectively.

8.8.4.2 Letrozole

Letrozole is an aromatase inhibitor of the enzyme that converts androgens to estrogens leading to an increase in FSH secretion and maturation of the ovarian follicle. Recent data suggested letrozole as the first-line therapy over clomiphene citrate for ovulation induction in women with PCOS and anovulatory infertility [24]. Importantly, a recent individual patient data meta-analysis showed that letrozole leads to higher ovulation [relative risk (RR) 1.13, 95% CI 1.07–1.2], clinical pregnancy (RR 1.45, 95% CI 1.23–1.70), and live birth rates (RR 1.43, 95% CI 1.17–1.75), as well as decreased time to pregnancy (hazard ratio 1.72, 95% CI

1.38–2.15), compared with clomiphene citrate [87]. In addition, the risk of multiple pregnancies appears to be less with letrozole compared to clomiphene citrate.

8.8.4.3 Clomiphene Citrate

Clomiphene citrate is a selective estrogen-receptor modulator traditionally used for ovulation induction for over 40 years, primarily due to oligoovulation or anovulation. It leads to higher clinical pregnancy rates compared with placebo or no treatment [24]. It could be used in preference over metformin for ovulation induction in obese women with PCOS with anovulatory infertility. Clomiphene citrate is an oral, cheap drug with relatively few adverse effects. The risk of multiple pregnancies is increased, and, therefore, monitoring is needed.

8.8.4.4 Metformin

Metformin has been used alone to promote ovulation in women with PCOS and anovulatory infertility, although women should be informed that there are more effective ovulation induction agents. A recent meta-analysis (41 studies, 4,552 women) showed that metformin increases ovulation (OR 2.64, 95% CI 1.85–3.75), clinical pregnancy (OR 1.98, 95% CI 1.47–2.65), and live birth rates (OR 1.59, 95% CI 1.00–2.51) compared to placebo in women with PCOS [88]. Metformin is also used in combination with clomiphene citrate to improve ovulation, clinical pregnancy, live birth rates, and time to pregnancy in obese women with PCOS [24]. The addition of metformin to clomiphene citrate may also decrease the time to pregnancy in clomiphene citrate-resistant women with anovulatory infertility. Metformin is an oral, cheap drug, with gastrointestinal disorders being the most common adverse event.

8.8.4.5 Exogenous Gonadotropins

The administration of exogenous gonadotropins constitutes a second-line treatment for ovulation induction. Although women with PCOS are not GnRH deficient, pulsatile GnRH is moderately effective for ovulation induction. In one study of 41 patients undergoing 114 ovulation induction cycles, 56% of women ovulated, and 40% of ovulatory patients achieved pregnancy [89]. Ovulatory cycles were associated with lower BMI and fasting insulin, and higher baseline FSH concentrations. Another study of 225 women with PCOS treated with low-dose gonadotropins found ovulation and pregnancy rates of 72% and 45%, respectively [90]. Exogenous gonadotropin administration is a high-cost option with the need for intensive ultrasound monitoring due to increased risk of multiple pregnancies and ovarian hyperstimulation syndrome (OHSS).

8.8.4.6 Laparoscopic Ovarian Drilling

For women who do not respond to letrozole or clomiphene citrate, laparoscopic ovarian drilling is a surgical option for second-line treatment. Compared with gonadotropin therapy, ovarian drilling has similar efficacy but a lower risk of multiple pregnancies or OHSS. Disadvantages of ovarian drilling include surgical risk and potential intra-abdominal adhesion formation. Ovarian drilling likely reduces the ovarian secretion of androgens, increasing LH and FSH secretion. In this way, the ovary is more responsive to stimulation by endogenous gonadotropins favoring the growth of a dominant ovarian follicle and ovulation. Following ovarian drilling, ovulatory cycles occur in 80% of patients [91], and also the normalization of ovulatory function is continued for many years in most patients [92].

8.8.4.7   Assisted Reproduction Technology (ART)
ART should be used in the case of failure of other treatments to stimulate ovaries as the third-line therapy. In vitro fertilization (IVF) is effective for anovulatory women with PCOS, and multiple pregnancies can be diminished by single-embryo transfer. OHSS risk is high in PCOS women undergoing IVF, and metformin administration before or during the IVF cycles may reduce the risk [93]. A GnRH antagonist protocol is preferred in women with PCOS undergoing IVF over a GnRH agonist protocol to reduce the stimulation time, the gonadotropin dose, and the OHSS risk.

8.8.4.8   Other Treatments
The evidence for non-pharmacological treatments such as inositol is not strong, highlighting the need for further research [94].

8.9   PCOS in Adolescents

The following recommendations have been suggested for the diagnosis of PCOS in adolescent girls and young women within 8 years of menarche [24, 95, 96]:

• Clinical and/or biochemical hyperandrogenism
• Menstrual irregularity that persists for 1–2 years

Diagnostic criteria for PCOS in adolescents are problematic because menstrual irregularity and acne are common in normal adolescents. For adolescents who have PCOS features but do not meet the diagnostic criteria, the provisional diagnosis "at risk for PCOS" is suggested to be given, considering reassessment at or before full reproductivity maturity (8 years post-menarche).

Although PCOS accounts for approximately 85% of androgen excess in adolescent girls, several other conditions present with hyperandrogenism. NCCAH is the second most common (4.2%) cause of hyperandrogenism in adolescence.

PCOS should be considered in any adolescent girl with a complaint of hirsutism, treatment-resistant acne, menstrual irregularity, acanthosis nigricans, and/or obesity [97]. Importantly, about one-third of cases come to medical attention because of hirsutism or acanthosis nigricans before menstrual irregularity becomes apparent.

An abnormal degree of acne is suggested by moderate or severe comedonal acne (>10 facial lesions) in early puberty, moderate or severe inflammatory acne through the perimenarcheal years, or acne that is persistent and poorly responsive to topical dermatologic therapy [98]. Balding is an unusual manifestation of hyperandrogenism in adolescents.

Acanthosis nigricans may be the presenting complaint of PCOS patients [99]. It is usually accompanied by obesity and may precede the onset of classical PCOS symptoms [97]. Although obesity is commonly associated with PCOS, it is not essential for the diagnosis because approximately one-half of patients are nonobese. Central obesity is common and is defined by a waist circumference of ≥88 cm in adolescents and adult women [100].

Importantly, ultrasound should not be used for PCOS diagnosis in those <8 years after menarche due to the high incidence of multi-follicular ovaries.

COCs use should be considered in adolescents with PCOS or at risk for PCOS to manage clinical hyperandrogenism and/or menstrual irregularity. Furthermore, in addition to lifestyle, metformin could be used in adolescent girls with PCOS or at risk for PCOS. Finally, COCs combined with metformin could be considered in overweight or obese adolescents with PCOS when COCs and lifestyle changes do not achieve the desired goals.

8.10   PCOS in Postmenopausal Women

Establishing PCOS diagnosis in postmenopausal women is problematic, but a possible diagnosis can be based upon a well-documented long-term history of oligomenorrhea and hyperandrogenism in the reproductive years [23]. PCOS morphology on ultrasound would provide additional support. However, ovarian volume and follicle number decrease with age in women with or without PCOS. Women with PCOS sometimes develop more regular menstrual cycles as they age [101], probably due to the age-dependent decrease in serum androgens and follicle count [102, 103].

8.11   Discussion and Future Perspectives

PCOS is a common endocrine disorder in women of reproductive age. It is associated with several health risks, including obesity, T2DM, cardiovascular disease, endometrial cancer, and mental health problems leading to a diminished quality of life. Lifelong care is needed, and it should be individualized based on the woman's risk profile, needs, concerns, and treatment goals. Lifestyle changes and weight loss remain the most important steps in PCOS management, with the choice of pharmacological treatment depending on fertility or non-fertility indications. Education of health professionals and screening of the disorder are needed for earlier diagnosis and subsequently effective intervention and prevention of the related health risks. Additionally, large sample studies are needed to deepen the understanding and the missing heritability of the syndrome and to evaluate the efficacy and safety of the different treatment options.

References

1. Bozdag G, Mumusoglu S, Zengin D, Karabulut E, Yildiz BO. The prevalence and phenotypic features of polycystic ovary syndrome: a systematic review and meta-analysis. Hum Reprod. 2016;31(12):2841–55.
2. Azziz R, Marin C, Hoq L, Badamgarav E, Song P. Health care-related economic burden of the polycystic ovary syndrome during the reproductive life span. J Clin Endocrinol Metab. 2005;90(8):4650–8.
3. Vink JM, Sadrzadeh S, Lambalk CB, Boomsma DI. Heritability of polycystic ovary syndrome in a Dutch twin-family study. J Clin Endocrinol Metab. 2006;91(6):2100–4.
4. Legro RS, Driscoll D, Strauss JF 3rd, Fox J, Dunaif A. Evidence for a genetic basis for hyperandrogenemia in polycystic ovary syndrome. Proc Natl Acad Sci U S A. 1998;95(25):14956–60.
5. Kahsar-Miller MD, Nixon C, Boots LR, Go RC, Azziz R. Prevalence of polycystic ovary syndrome (PCOS) in first-degree relatives of patients with PCOS. Fertil Steril. 2001;75(1):53–8.
6. Hiam D, Moreno-Asso A, Teede HJ, Laven JSE, Stepto NK, Moran LJ, et al. The genetics of polycystic ovary syndrome: an overview of candidate gene systematic reviews and genome-wide association studies. J Clin Med. 2019;8(10):1606.
7. Crespo RP, Bachega T, Mendonca BB, Gomes LG. An update of genetic basis of PCOS pathogenesis. Arch Endocrinol Metab. 2018;62(3):352–61.
8. Xita N, Tsatsoulis A. Review: fetal programming of polycystic ovary syndrome by androgen excess: evidence from experimental, clinical, and genetic association studies. J Clin Endocrinol Metab. 2006;91(5):1660–6.
9. Rutkowska AZ, Diamanti-Kandarakis E. Polycystic ovary syndrome and environmental toxins. Fertil Steril. 2016;106(4):948–58.
10. Balen AH. Hypersecretion of luteinizing hormone and the polycystic ovary syndrome. Hum Reprod. 1993;8(Suppl 2):123–8.
11. Waldstreicher J, Santoro NF, Hall JE, Filicori M, Crowley WF Jr. Hyperfunction of the hypothalamic-pituitary axis in women with polycystic ovarian disease: indirect evidence for partial gonadotroph desensitization. J Clin Endocrinol Metab. 1988;66(1):165–72.
12. Jakimiuk AJ, Weitsman SR, Navab A, Magoffin DA. Luteinizing hormone receptor, steroidogenesis acute regulatory protein, and steroidogenic enzyme messenger ribonucleic acids are overexpressed in thecal and granulosa cells from polycystic ovaries. J Clin Endocrinol Metab. 2001;86(3):1318–23.
13. Taylor AE, McCourt B, Martin KA, Anderson EJ, Adams JM, Schoenfeld D, et al. Determinants of abnormal gonadotropin secretion in clinically defined women with polycystic ovary syndrome. J Clin Endocrinol Metab. 1997;82(7):2248–56.
14. Goodarzi MO, Carmina E, Azziz R. DHEA, DHEAS and PCOS. J Steroid Biochem Mol Biol. 2015;145:213–25.
15. Burt Solorzano CM, McCartney CR, Blank SK, Knudsen KL, Marshall JC. Hyperandrogenaemia in adolescent girls: origins of abnormal gonadotropin-releasing hormone secretion. BJOG. 2010;117(2):143–9.
16. Broekmans FJ, Visser JA, Laven JS, Broer SL, Themmen AP, Fauser BC. Anti-Mullerian hormone and ovarian dysfunction. Trends Endocrinol Metab. 2008;19(9):340–7.
17. Dunaif A. Insulin resistance and the polycystic ovary syndrome: mechanism and implications for pathogenesis. Endocr Rev. 1997;18(6):774–800.
18. Diamanti-Kandarakis E, Dunaif A. Insulin resistance and the polycystic ovary syndrome revisited: an update on mechanisms and implications. Endocr Rev. 2012;33(6):981–1030.
19. Dunaif A, Xia J, Book CB, Schenker E, Tang Z. Excessive insulin receptor serine phosphorylation in cultured fibroblasts and in skeletal muscle. A potential mechanism for insulin resistance in the polycystic ovary syndrome. J Clin Invest. 1995;96(2):801–10.
20. Nestler JE, Jakubowicz DJ, de Vargas AF, Brik C, Quintero N, Medina F. Insulin stimulates testosterone biosynthesis by human thecal cells from women with polycystic ovary syndrome by activating its own receptor and using inositolglycan mediators as the signal transduction system. J Clin Endocrinol Metab. 1998;83(6):2001–5.

21. Nestler JE, Powers LP, Matt DW, Steingold KA, Plymate SR, Rittmaster RS, et al. A direct effect of hyperinsulinemia on serum sex hormone-binding globulin levels in obese women with the polycystic ovary syndrome. J Clin Endocrinol Metab. 1991;72(1):83–9.
22. Rotterdam ESHRE/ASRM-Sponsored PCOS Consensus Workshop Group. Revised 2003 consensus on diagnostic criteria and long-term health risks related to polycystic ovary syndrome (PCOS). Hum Reprod. 2004;19(1):41–7.
23. Legro RS, Arslanian SA, Ehrmann DA, Hoeger KM, Murad MH, Pasquali R, et al. Diagnosis and treatment of polycystic ovary syndrome: an Endocrine Society clinical practice guideline. J Clin Endocrinol Metab. 2013;98(12):4565–92.
24. Teede HJ, Misso ML, Costello MF, Dokras A, Laven J, Moran L, et al. Recommendations from the international evidence-based guideline for the assessment and management of polycystic ovary syndrome. Fertil Steril. 2018;110(3):364–79.
25. Azziz R, Carmina E, Dewailly D, Diamanti-Kandarakis E, Escobar-Morreale HF, Futterweit W, et al. The Androgen Excess and PCOS Society criteria for the polycystic ovary syndrome: the complete task force report. Fertil Steril. 2009;91(2):456–88.
26. Zawadski J, Dunaif A. Diagnostic criteria for polycystic ovary syndrome: towards a rational approach. In: Dunaif A, Givens J, Haseltine FP, Merriam GE, editors. Polycystic ovary syndrome. Current issues in endocrinology and metabolism. Boston: Blackwell Scientific Inc.; 1992. p. 377.
27. Boyle JA, Cunningham J, O'Dea K, Dunbar T, Norman RJ. Prevalence of polycystic ovary syndrome in a sample of Indigenous women in Darwin, Australia. Med J Aust. 2012;196(1):62–6.
28. Lizneva D, Suturina L, Walker W, Brakta S, Gavrilova-Jordan L, Azziz R. Criteria, prevalence, and phenotypes of polycystic ovary syndrome. Fertil Steril. 2016;106(1):6–15.
29. Munro MG, Critchley HOD, Fraser IS, Committee FMD. The two FIGO systems for normal and abnormal uterine bleeding symptoms and classification of causes of abnormal uterine bleeding in the reproductive years: 2018 revisions. Int J Gynaecol Obstet. 2018;143(3):393–408.
30. Martin KA, Anderson RR, Chang RJ, Ehrmann DA, Lobo RA, Murad MH, et al. Evaluation and treatment of hirsutism in premenopausal women: an Endocrine Society clinical practice guideline. J Clin Endocrinol Metab. 2018;103(4):1233–57.
31. Hatch R, Rosenfield RL, Kim MH, Tredway D. Hirsutism: implications, etiology, and management. Am J Obstet Gynecol. 1981;140(7):815–30.
32. Escobar-Morreale HF, Carmina E, Dewailly D, Gambineri A, Kelestimur F, Moghetti P, et al. Epidemiology, diagnosis and management of hirsutism: a consensus statement by the Androgen Excess and Polycystic Ovary Syndrome Society. Hum Reprod Update. 2012;18(2):146–70.
33. Yildiz BO. Diagnosis of hyperandrogenism: clinical criteria. Best Pract Res Clin Endocrinol Metab. 2006;20(2):167–76.
34. Carmina E, Azziz R, Bergfeld W, Escobar-Morreale HF, Futterweit W, Huddleston H, et al. Female pattern hair loss and androgen excess: a report from the multidisciplinary androgen excess and PCOS Committee. J Clin Endocrinol Metab. 2019;104(7):2875–91.
35. Laven JS, Mulders AG, Visser JA, Themmen AP, De Jong FH, Fauser BC. Anti-Mullerian hormone serum concentrations in normoovulatory and anovulatory women of reproductive age. J Clin Endocrinol Metab. 2004;89(1):318–23.
36. Iliodromiti S, Kelsey TW, Anderson RA, Nelson SM. Can anti-Mullerian hormone predict the diagnosis of polycystic ovary syndrome? A systematic review and meta-analysis of extracted data. J Clin Endocrinol Metab. 2013;98(8):3332–40.
37. Dumont A, Robin G, Catteau-Jonard S, Dewailly D. Role of Anti-Mullerian Hormone in pathophysiology, diagnosis and treatment of Polycystic Ovary Syndrome: a review. Reprod Biol Endocrinol. 2015;13:137.
38. Kaltsas GA, Korbonits M, Isidori AM, Webb JA, Trainer PJ, Monson JP, et al. How common are polycystic ovaries and the polycystic ovarian syndrome in women with Cushing's syndrome? Clin Endocrinol (Oxf). 2000;53(4):493–500.

39. Kaltsas GA, Mukherjee JJ, Jenkins PJ, Satta MA, Islam N, Monson JP, et al. Menstrual irregularity in women with acromegaly. J Clin Endocrinol Metab. 1999;84(8):2731–5.
40. Derksen J, Nagesser SK, Meinders AE, Haak HR, van de Velde CJ. Identification of virilizing adrenal tumors in hirsute women. N Engl J Med. 1994;331(15):968–73.
41. The Amsterdam ESHRE/ASRM-Sponsored 3rd PCOS Consensus Workshop Group. Consensus on women's health aspects of polycystic ovary syndrome (PCOS). Hum Reprod. 2012;27:14–24.
42. Quinonez Zarza C, Silva Ruiz R, Torres Juarez JM. [Obesity, arterial hypertension, metabolic disorders, and polycystic ovary syndrome]. Ginecol Obstet Mex. 2000;68:317–22.
43. Azziz R, Sanchez LA, Knochenhauer ES, Moran C, Lazenby J, Stephens KC, et al. Androgen excess in women: experience with over 1000 consecutive patients. J Clin Endocrinol Metab. 2004;89(2):453–62.
44. Hedley AA, Ogden CL, Johnson CL, Carroll MD, Curtin LR, Flegal KM. Prevalence of overweight and obesity among US children, adolescents, and adults, 1999-2002. JAMA. 2004;291(23):2847–50.
45. Carmina E, Rosato F, Janni A, Rizzo M, Longo RA. Extensive clinical experience: relative prevalence of different androgen excess disorders in 950 women referred because of clinical hyperandrogenism. J Clin Endocrinol Metab. 2006;91(1):2–6.
46. Ehrmann DA, Barnes RB, Rosenfield RL, Cavaghan MK, Imperial J. Prevalence of impaired glucose tolerance and diabetes in women with polycystic ovary syndrome. Diabetes Care. 1999;22(1):141–6.
47. Ehrmann DA, Kasza K, Azziz R, Legro RS, Ghazzi MN, PCOS/Troglitazone Study Group. Effects of race and family history of type 2 diabetes on metabolic status of women with poly-cystic ovary syndrome. J Clin Endocrinol Metab. 2005;90(1):66–71.
48. Legro RS, Gnatuk CL, Kunselman AR, Dunaif A. Changes in glucose tolerance over time in women with polycystic ovary syndrome: a controlled study. J Clin Endocrinol Metab. 2005;90(6):3236–42.
49. Wild RA, Rizzo M, Clifton S, Carmina E. Lipid levels in polycystic ovary syndrome: system-atic review and meta-analysis. Fertil Steril. 2011;95(3):1073-9.e1–11.
50. Legro RS, Azziz R, Ehrmann D, Fereshetian AG, O'Keefe M, Ghazzi MN. Minimal response of circulating lipids in women with polycystic ovary syndrome to improvement in insulin sensitivity with troglitazone. J Clin Endocrinol Metab. 2003;88(11):5137–44.
51. Dunaif A, Segal KR, Futterweit W, Dobrjansky A. Profound peripheral insulin resistance, independent of obesity, in polycystic ovary syndrome. Diabetes. 1989;38(9):1165–74.
52. DeUgarte CM, Bartolucci AA, Azziz R. Prevalence of insulin resistance in the polycystic ovary syndrome using the homeostasis model assessment. Fertil Steril. 2005;83(5):1454–60.
53. Wild RA, Carmina E, Diamanti-Kandarakis E, Dokras A, Escobar-Morreale HF, Futterweit W, et al. Assessment of cardiovascular risk and prevention of cardiovascular disease in women with the polycystic ovary syndrome: a consensus statement by the Androgen Excess and Polycystic Ovary Syndrome (AE-PCOS) Society. J Clin Endocrinol Metab. 2010;95(5):2038–49.
54. Ford ES, Giles WH, Mokdad AH. Increasing prevalence of the metabolic syndrome among U.S. Adults. Diabetes Care. 2004;27(10):2444–9.
55. Apridonidze T, Essah PA, Iuorno MJ, Nestler JE. Prevalence and characteristics of the metabolic syndrome in women with polycystic ovary syndrome. J Clin Endocrinol Metab. 2005;90(4):1929–35.
56. Setji TL, Holland ND, Sanders LL, Pereira KC, Diehl AM, Brown AJ. Nonalcoholic steato-hepatitis and nonalcoholic Fatty liver disease in young women with polycystic ovary syn-drome. J Clin Endocrinol Metab. 2006;91(5):1741–7.
57. Cerda C, Perez-Ayuso RM, Riquelme A, Soza A, Villaseca P, Sir-Petermann T, et al. Nonalcoholic fatty liver disease in women with polycystic ovary syndrome. J Hepatol. 2007;47(3):412–7.
58. Simon S, Rahat H, Carreau AM, Garcia-Reyes Y, Halbower A, Pyle L, et al. Poor sleep is related to metabolic syndrome severity in adolescents with PCOS and obesity. J Clin Endocrinol Metab. 2020;105(4):e1827.

59. Vgontzas AN, Legro RS, Bixler EO, Grayev A, Kales A, Chrousos GP. Polycystic ovary syndrome is associated with obstructive sleep apnea and daytime sleepiness: role of insulin resistance. J Clin Endocrinol Metab. 2001;86(2):517–20.
60. Tasali E, Van Cauter E, Hoffman L, Ehrmann DA. Impact of obstructive sleep apnea on insulin resistance and glucose tolerance in women with polycystic ovary syndrome. J Clin Endocrinol Metab. 2008;93(10):3878–84.
61. Lo JC, Feigenbaum SL, Yang J, Pressman AR, Selby JV, Go AS. Epidemiology and adverse cardiovascular risk profile of diagnosed polycystic ovary syndrome. J Clin Endocrinol Metab. 2006;91(4):1357–63.
62. Wild RA. Polycystic ovary syndrome: a risk for coronary artery disease? Am J Obstet Gynecol. 2002;186(1):35–43.
63. Toulis KA, Goulis DG, Mintziori G, Kintiraki E, Eukarpidis E, Mouratoglou SA, et al. Meta-analysis of cardiovascular disease risk markers in women with polycystic ovary syndrome. Hum Reprod Update. 2011;17(6):741–60.
64. de Groot PC, Dekkers OM, Romijn JA, Dieben SW, Helmerhorst FM. PCOS, coronary heart disease, stroke and the influence of obesity: a systematic review and meta-analysis. Hum Reprod Update. 2011;17(4):495–500.
65. Shafiee MN, Khan G, Ariffin R, Abu J, Chapman C, Deen S, et al. Preventing endometrial cancer risk in polycystic ovarian syndrome (PCOS) women: could metformin help? Gynecol Oncol. 2014;132(1):248–53.
66. Giudice LC. Endometrium in PCOS: implantation and predisposition to endocrine CA. Best Pract Res Clin Endocrinol Metab. 2006;20(2):235–44.
67. Barry JA, Azizia MM, Hardiman PJ. Risk of endometrial, ovarian and breast cancer in women with polycystic ovary syndrome: a systematic review and meta-analysis. Hum Reprod Update. 2014;20(5):748–58.
68. Cheung AP. Ultrasound and menstrual history in predicting endometrial hyperplasia in polycystic ovary syndrome. Obstet Gynecol. 2001;98(2):325–31.
69. Glueck CJ, Wang P, Goldenberg N, Sieve-Smith L. Pregnancy outcomes among women with polycystic ovary syndrome treated with metformin. Hum Reprod. 2002;17(11):2858–64.
70. Qin JZ, Pang LH, Li MJ, Fan XJ, Huang RD, Chen HY. Obstetric complications in women with polycystic ovary syndrome: a systematic review and meta-analysis. Reprod Biol Endocrinol. 2013;11:56.
71. Palomba S, Falbo A, Chiossi G, Orio F, Tolino A, Colao A, et al. Low-grade chronic inflammation in pregnant women with polycystic ovary syndrome: a prospective controlled clinical study. J Clin Endocrinol Metab. 2014;99(8):2942–51.
72. Bhattacharya SM, Jha A. Prevalence and risk of depressive disorders in women with polycystic ovary syndrome (PCOS). Fertil Steril. 2010;94(1):357–9.
73. Dokras A, Stener-Victorin E, Yildiz BO, Li R, Ottey S, Shah D, et al. Androgen Excess-Polycystic Ovary Syndrome Society: position statement on depression, anxiety, quality of life, and eating disorders in polycystic ovary syndrome. Fertil Steril. 2018;109(5):888–99.
74. Naessen S, Carlstrom K, Garoff L, Glant R, Hirschberg AL. Polycystic ovary syndrome in bulimic women—an evaluation based on the new diagnostic criteria. Gynecol Endocrinol. 2006;22(7):388–94.
75. Pasquali R, Gambineri A, Cavazza C, Ibarra Gasparini D, Ciampaglia W, Cognigni GE, et al. Heterogeneity in the responsiveness to long-term lifestyle intervention and predictability in obese women with polycystic ovary syndrome. Eur J Endocrinol. 2011;164(1):53–60.
76. Lamos EM, Malek R, Davis SN. GLP-1 receptor agonists in the treatment of polycystic ovary syndrome. Expert Rev Clin Pharmacol. 2017;10(4):401–8.
77. Escobar-Morreale HF, Botella-Carretero JI, Alvarez-Blasco F, Sancho J, San Millan JL. The polycystic ovary syndrome associated with morbid obesity may resolve after weight loss induced by bariatric surgery. J Clin Endocrinol Metab. 2005;90(12):6364–9.

78. Moran LJ, Tassone EC, Boyle J, Brennan L, Harrison CL, Hirschberg AL, et al. Evidence summaries and recommendations from the international evidence-based guideline for the assessment and management of polycystic ovary syndrome: lifestyle management. Obes Rev. 2020;21(10):e13046.

79. Ortega-Gonzalez C, Luna S, Hernandez L, Crespo G, Aguayo P, Arteaga-Troncoso G, et al. Responses of serum androgen and insulin resistance to metformin and pioglitazone in obese, insulin-resistant women with polycystic ovary syndrome. J Clin Endocrinol Metab. 2005;90(3):1360–5.

80. Brettenthaler N, De Geyter C, Huber PR, Keller U. Effect of the insulin sensitizer pioglitazone on insulin resistance, hyperandrogenism, and ovulatory dysfunction in women with polycystic ovary syndrome. J Clin Endocrinol Metab. 2004;89(8):3835–40.

81. Pasquali R, Antenucci D, Casimirri F, Venturoli S, Paradisi R, Fabbri R, et al. Clinical and hormonal characteristics of obese amenorrheic hyperandrogenic women before and after weight loss. J Clin Endocrinol Metab. 1989;68(1):173–9.

82. Kiddy DS, Hamilton-Fairley D, Bush A, Short F, Anyaoku V, Reed MJ, et al. Improvement in endocrine and ovarian function during dietary treatment of obese women with polycystic ovary syndrome. Clin Endocrinol (Oxf). 1992;36(1):105–11.

83. Oguz SH, Yildiz BO. An update on contraception in polycystic ovary syndrome. Endocrinol Metab (Seoul). 2021;36(2):296–311.

84. Roach RE, Helmerhorst FM, Lijfering WM, Stijnen T, Algra A, Dekkers OM. Combined oral contraceptives: the risk of myocardial infarction and ischemic stroke. Cochrane Database Syst Rev. 2015;(8):CD011054.

85. Moghetti P, Castello R, Negri C, Tosi F, Perrone F, Caputo M, et al. Metformin effects on clinical features, endocrine and metabolic profiles, and insulin sensitivity in polycystic ovary syndrome: a randomized, double-blind, placebo-controlled 6-month trial, followed by open, long-term clinical evaluation. J Clin Endocrinol Metab. 2000;85(1):139–46.

86. The Thessaloniki ESHRE/ASRM-Sponsored PCOS Consensus Workshop Group. Consensus on infertility treatment related to polycystic ovary syndrome. Fertil Steril. 2008;89(3):505–22.

87. Wang R, Li W, Bordewijk EM, Legro RS, Zhang H, Wu X, et al. First-line ovulation induction for polycystic ovary syndrome: an individual participant data meta-analysis. Hum Reprod Update. 2019;25(6):717–32.

88. Sharpe A, Morley LC, Tang T, Norman RJ, Balen AH. Metformin for ovulation induction (excluding gonadotrophins) in women with polycystic ovary syndrome. Cochrane Database Syst Rev. 2019;12:CD013505.

89. Gill S, Taylor AE, Martin KA, Welt CK, Adams JM, Hall JE. Specific factors predict the response to pulsatile gonadotropin-releasing hormone therapy in polycystic ovarian syndrome. J Clin Endocrinol Metab. 2001;86(6):2428–36.

90. White DM, Polson DW, Kiddy D, Sagle P, Watson H, Gilling-Smith C, et al. Induction of ovulation with low-dose gonadotropins in polycystic ovary syndrome: an analysis of 109 pregnancies in 225 women. J Clin Endocrinol Metab. 1996;81(11):3821–4.

91. Seow KM, Juan CC, Hwang JL, Ho LT. Laparoscopic surgery in polycystic ovary syndrome: reproductive and metabolic effects. Semin Reprod Med. 2008;26(1):101–10.

92. Amer SA, Banu Z, Li TC, Cooke ID. Long-term follow-up of patients with polycystic ovary syndrome after laparoscopic ovarian drilling: endocrine and ultrasonographic outcomes. Hum Reprod. 2002;17(11):2851–7.

93. Tso LO, Costello MF, Albuquerque LE, Andriolo RB, Freitas V. Metformin treatment before and during IVF or ICSI in women with polycystic ovary syndrome. Cochrane Database Syst Rev. 2009;(2):CD006105.

94. Pundir J, Charles D, Sabatini L, Hiam D, Jitpiriyaroj S, Teede H, et al. Overview of systematic reviews of non-pharmacological interventions in women with polycystic ovary syndrome. Hum Reprod Update. 2019;25(2):243–56.

95. Witchel SF, Oberfield S, Rosenfield RL, Codner E, Bonny A, Ibanez L, et al. The diagnosis of polycystic ovary syndrome during adolescence. Horm Res Paediatr. 2015. Apr 1. https://doi.org/10.1159/000375530. Online ahead of print.
96. Ibanez L, Oberfield SE, Witchel S, Auchus RJ, Chang RJ, Codner E, et al. An international consortium update: pathophysiology, diagnosis, and treatment of polycystic ovarian syndrome in adolescence. Horm Res Paediatr. 2017;88(6):371–95.
97. Rosenfield RL, Ehrmann DA, Littlejohn EE. Adolescent polycystic ovary syndrome due to functional ovarian hyperandrogenism persists into adulthood. J Clin Endocrinol Metab. 2015;100(4):1537–43.
98. Eichenfield LF, Krakowski AC, Piggott C, Del Rosso J, Baldwin H, Friedlander SF, et al. Evidence-based recommendations for the diagnosis and treatment of pediatric acne. Pediatrics. 2013;131(Suppl 3):S163–86.
99. Dunaif A, Green G, Phelps RG, Lebwohl M, Futterweit W, Lewy L. Acanthosis Nigricans, insulin action, and hyperandrogenism: clinical, histological, and biochemical findings. J Clin Endocrinol Metab. 1991;73(3):590–5.
100. Leibel NI, Baumann EE, Kocherginsky M, Rosenfield RL. Relationship of adolescent polycystic ovary syndrome to parental metabolic syndrome. J Clin Endocrinol Metab. 2006;91(4):1275–83.
101. Elting MW, Korsen TJ, Rekers-Mombarg LT, Schoemaker J. Women with polycystic ovary syndrome gain regular menstrual cycles when ageing. Hum Reprod. 2000;15(1):24–8.
102. Winters SJ, Talbott E, Guzick DS, Zborowski J, McHugh KP. Serum testosterone levels decrease in middle age in women with the polycystic ovary syndrome. Fertil Steril. 2000;73(4):724–9.
103. Elting MW, Kwee J, Korsen TJ, Rekers-Mombarg LT, Schoemaker J. Aging women with polycystic ovary syndrome who achieve regular menstrual cycles have a smaller follicle cohort than those who continue to have irregular cycles. Fertil Steril. 2003;79(5):1154–60.

Amenorrhea Associated with Contraception and the Postpartum Period

9

Alice Antonelli, Andrea Giannini, Tiziana Fidecicchi,
Marisa Ardito, Andrea R. Genazzani, Tommaso Simoncini,
and Merki-Feld Gabriele

9.1   Introduction

Close or unplanned pregnancies represent a risk to both mother and child. Spacing pregnancies at least 2 years apart can prevent 30% of maternal deaths, 10% of infant deaths, and 20% of deaths between 1 and 4 years of age [1]. A recent Canadian cohort study of nearly 150,000 pregnancies reported both increased maternal mortality and risks of serious morbidity in women 35 years of age or older with short interpregnancy interval (IPI). However, women aged 20–34 years with short IPI had a higher risk of adverse fetal and infant outcomes [2].

An IPI shorter than 18 months between delivery and subsequent conception exposes women to an increased risk of preterm birth, low birth weight, and small-for-gestational age (SGA) infants. A retrospective cohort study of more than 69,000 women in Scotland using population-based registers from the 1990s found that a short interval (less than 6 months) between term delivery of a newborn and initiation of a new pregnancy is an independent risk factor for subsequent preterm delivery, neonatal death not due to malformations, or Rh incompatibility; however, for intrauterine death from unknown causes, the increased risk is not statistically significant [3]. Conversely, subjects receiving contraception have a significantly lower risk of unintended pregnancy and short IPI [4]. Worldwide, contraception prevents 30% of maternal

A. Antonelli · A. Giannini · T. Fidecicchi · M. Ardito · T. Simoncini
Division of Obstetrics and Gynecology, Department of Experimental and Clinical Medicine,
University of Pisa, Pisa, Italy
e-mail: alice.antonelli@unipi.it; andrea.giannini@unipi.it; tommaso.simoncini@unipi.it

A. R. Genazzani
International Society of Gynecological Endocrinology, Pisa, Italy

M.-F. Gabriele (✉)
Clinic of Reproductive Endocrinology, University of Zurich, Zurich, Switzerland
e-mail: Gabriele.Merki@usz.ch

© International Society of Gynecological Endocrinology 2023
A. R. Genazzani et al. (eds.), *Amenorrhea*, ISGE Series,
https://doi.org/10.1007/978-3-031-22378-5_9

mortality and 10% of infant deaths if pregnancies are spaced 2 years apart [5]. Therefore, the World Health Organization from a global perspective recommends an interval of at least 24 months between birth and subsequent conception in order to reduce the risks of maternal, perinatal, and infant adverse outcomes.

Demographic surveys in developing countries indicate that 95% of women would like to avoid pregnancy for at least 2 years, but 65% of them do not use contraception because they cannot afford it [6]. In sub-Saharan Africa, this percentage rises to 75% of postpartum women. Obviously, these numbers are much better in industrialized countries, which nevertheless maintain ranges that vary to a greater or lesser degree between north and south. The contraceptive needs of women in the postpartum period are probably underestimated. It is possible that sexual activity and fertility begin early while, on the other hand, the needs of caring for the newborn may constitute a specific obstacle to access an effective contraceptive method. For this reason, effective contraception should be offered to all women, whether or not they are breastfeeding, as soon as possible and no later than 21 days after delivery. For this purpose, adequate information helps each mother and couple to better plan their fertility. The British guidelines, for example, in the document "Contraception After Pregnancy" by the Faculty of Family Planning and Reproductive Health Care Clinical Effectiveness Unit (FSRH) [7], recommend that the issue of contraception be discussed continuously in services dedicated to perinatal care: during pregnancy (to allow women to make a timely choice after delivery), but also in peripartum and postpartum care. Such information is desirable for all mothers, especially adolescent mothers, to whom it is advisable to recommend a long-acting reversible contraception (LARC) method. LARCs include the IUD-CU, the IUS-LNG, subcutaneous implants, pills without interruption, and intramuscular injections of medroxyprogesterone acetate.

During counselling, the doctor must assess the specific contraceptive needs in relation to personal choices in terms of family fertility; sexual activity more or less present/frequent; time passed since delivery; return or not of menstruation; type of breastfeeding (exclusive or not); social (such as resumption of work), cultural, or religious factors; previous experience with contraceptive methods; lifestyle (smoking); and also medical factors (risk of thromboembolism, previous thromboembolism, hypertension, diabetes, previous trophoblastic disease, liver disease, current medications, etc.) [8]. During the consultation, the inhibitory potential on ovulation by the baby's sucking rhythms, which varies as the months progress, should be assessed.

9.2 Breastfeeding Effects on Ovulation

The woman should be informed that breastfeeding delays the resumption of ovulation, both because of the persistence of high prolactin levels and because suction modifies gonadotropin pulsatility [9]. For this reason, all the contraceptive methods used have a lower number of failures than in other moments of the fertile life. However, the reduction in the number of suctions is followed by an increase in ovulatory possibilities. In women who do not breastfeed, ovulation can occur approximately 1 or 2 months after childbirth, while in those who breastfeed, ovulation can occur as early as 3 months after childbirth. According to the Bellagio Conference in 1988, all bleedings in the first 56 days after delivery should not be considered as the end of amenorrhea. In 1996, Labbok et al. defined menstruation as two continuous days of vaginal bleeding that the woman considered similar to a menstrual period or heavier, or two continuous days of spotting and one day of bleeding, or three continuous days of spotting [10]. In 1999, the World Health Organization used four different definitions as the end of amenorrhea. A Cochrane review published in 2015 proposed to redefine amenorrhea as no vaginal bleeding for at least 10 days after the end of postpartum bleeding [11]. The incidence of real menstruation at 6 months evaluated with life tables in 13 studies varied from 11.1 to 39.4% [12]. Prospective studies have shown that the return of menstruation occurs on average 28 weeks after delivery in women who breastfeed [13]. If menstruation is also combined with ovulation, the woman is at risk for an unwanted pregnancy.

9.3   Counselling

Decisions about birth spacing are informed by multiple factors, including desired family size, beliefs about and access to contraception, and maternal age. Furthermore, the postpartum period is a clinically dynamic time, in which method eligibility may change based on venous thromboembolism (VTE) risk, breastfeeding status, and medical comorbidities. Women often have a clear plan for postpartum contraception if counselling is done during the prenatal period, which then allows clinicians to ensure that the desired method is available after delivery. Eliciting a discussion of a woman's reproductive life plan is a natural start to counselling regarding postpartum contraception. This conversation should include questions about desire for, and timing of, any future pregnancies and should begin during prenatal care [14]. Once the woman's desire for additional children and subsequent birth spacing has been established, the clinicians need to determine the contraceptive characteristics that she values most at that time, including efficacy, convenience (both in obtaining and using the method), cost, ability to control whether to use the method, effect on uterine bleeding, and compatibility with breastfeeding [15].

9.4   Contraceptive Methods (Table 9.1)

The contraceptive methods that can be used are surgical (sterilization), barrier (male or female condom), chemical, mechanical (IUD-Cu), hormonal (oral contraception, patch, ring, POP, IUS-LNG, subcutaneous implant, injectable), and natural. Each method has indications, contraindications, advantages, and disadvantages in its postpartum use, both in women who are breastfeeding and those who are not. From a practical point of view, the use of contraceptive methods in specific biological or clinical conditions implies a certain category of risk that affects their use as indicated by the WHO [16]. Each method has a precise time in the postpartum in which we can assume the beginning of the assumption with a good degree of safety [17] (Table 9.2).

Table 9.1 Birth control method failure rates and efficacy

Contraceptive method	Adjusted pearl index (perfect use failure rate)	Pearl index (typical use failure rate)	Efficacy (%) (perfect use)
Progestin intrauterine device (IUD)	0.5	0.7	>99
Copper IUD	0.6	0.8	>99
Combined oral contraceptive—the pill	0.3	7	>99
Progestin-only pill—mini-pills	0.3	7	>99
Progestogen-only injection	0.2	4	>99
Monthly injection or combined injectable contraceptive (CIC)	0.05	3	>99
Vaginal ring	0.3	7	>99
Contraceptive patch	0.3	7	>99
Hormone implant or rod	0.1	0.1	>99
Sponge	9—women that have never had children 20—women that have had children	12—women that have never had children 24—women that have had children	80–91
Diaphragm	4–8	12	92–96
Male condom	2	13	98
Female condom	5	21	95
Cervical cap	4–8	17–23	92–96
Chemical contraceptives—spermicides	18	28	82
Withdrawal (coitus interruptus)	4	20	96
No contraception	85	85	15
Sterilization of the woman	0.5	0.5	>99
Sterilization of the man	0.1	0.15	>99
Calendar method	Unknown	15–24	

Table 9.2 Time to start a contraceptive method in postpartum breastfeeding woman

Time after delivery	Method
Immediate	Male and female condom
	LAM
	IUD-Cu
	Tubal sterilization during cesarean section
Within 4 weeks	POP
	Subcutaneous etonogestrel implantation
	Emergency contraception with LNG
From 4 weeks onwards	IUD-Cu
	IUS-LNG
6 weeks and after	COC
	Diaphragm
	Laparoscopic tubal sterilization

9.4.1   Lactational Amenorrhea Method (LAM)

The lactational amenorrhea method [18] has been included in many educational programs in various parts of the world and is used by several hundred million women. The necessity to learn, start, and continue the LAM method is particularly evident in developing countries, where for cultural and socioeconomic reasons, the duration of the breastfeeding period is much longer than in developed countries. There are three prerequisites that must be fulfilled in order to adhere to the LAM method: the patient must be in her first 6 months after childbirth, in a state of amenorrhea, and in exclusive breastfeeding with intervals between feedings never exceeding 6 h at night and 4 h during the day [19].

9.4.2   Surgical Methods

Surgical methods should be used in cases where the couple's reproductive plan is concluded or there are contraindications to the use of other methods. Obviously, they should be considered as a "presumably definitive" choice, excluding hysterectomy, which is "categorically definitive." The adverb "presumably" derives from at least two considerations: first, tubal sterilization is not 100% safe, particularly if performed during cesarean section or in the immediate postpartum period; second, because an attempt at recanalization can be performed successfully, albeit with low probability of success, with microsurgical techniques in cases of afterthought. Reconsideration, according to case histories, may occur in between 1 and 26% of cases, particularly in younger women [20]. Tubal sterilization may be performed during a cesarean section or in the immediate postpartum period. Some women couples choose a 24–48-h wait for evidence of normal physical condition of the newborn. During cesarean section, Pomeroy's technique is preferred, either classic (ligature with section and removal of the two tubal stumps) or modified (e.g., Madlener's technique, which involves tubal ligation only). Other similar procedures are sometimes performed (such as Parkland's or Irving's procedures). The woman should be adequately informed about possible reconsideration and chances of failure, which are around 1% at 10 years [21]. After a vaginal delivery, laparoscopic tubal sterilization with metal clips is preferred (techniques by Hulka or Filshie). Their safety is very high, with modest clinical commitment. Bipolar coagulation, which destroys part of the tube, is sometimes used. Recently, transcervical tubal sterilization has also entered clinical practice, using a hysteroscope that places a micro metal device in each of the two tubes. Not to forget the option of male sterilization (vasectomy).

9.4.3   Barrier Methods and Local Chemicals

Barrier methods (male and female condoms, vaginal diaphragm) have the great advantage of defending against sexually transmitted diseases and in any case do not affect the health of the mother or the child, since they have no systemic effects.

Male and female condoms can be freely used after childbirth at the first resumption of sexual activity. They do not affect lactation and can be used alongside other methods when the woman eventually uses them after abandoning LAM. The diaphragm requires that uterine and cervical involution be completed, which requires at least 6 weeks after delivery. In Italy, nowadays, this method is actually rather overused. Local spermicides (creams or ovules), usually containing 9-nonoxynol, are not very effective on their own. They should be used in association with a diaphragm, but there are also male condoms with added 9-nonoxynol that should be avoided in women who are at risk of sexually transmitted diseases [22].

9.4.4 Intrauterine Device (IUD)

Intrauterine devices provide highly effective contraception (CU-IUD; LNG-IUS) and are commonly placed at an interval postpartum visit typically 4–6 weeks after delivery for women who desire intrauterine contraception. Immediate postpartum IUD placement, within 10 min of delivery, is safe and effective; however, the risk of expulsion is greater among women receiving immediate IUDs compared with interval placement [23]. As for the risk of uterine perforation, it increases throughout lactation and is highest up to 6 months after delivery for both copper intrauterine devices and LNG-IUS.

The U.S. Medical Eligibility Criteria for Contraceptive Use supports the safety of IUD placement during this early time period [24].

9.5   Hormonal Therapies

9.5.1 Estroprogestinic (EP) Contraception

The use of oral estroprogestinic contraception should be carefully evaluated considering the increased postpartum venous thromboembolic risk. In particular, up to 6 weeks after birth, it should not be used when the following risk factors for deep vein thrombosis (DVT) are present: prolonged immobilization, hereditary thrombophilia, postpartum hemorrhage, BMI >30, smoking, postpartum transfusion, preeclampsia, and cesarean section [7]. In other cases, combined estroprogestinic contraceptives can be assumed starting from the 21st day after childbirth if the woman is not breastfeeding, and not before 6 weeks after childbirth if the patient is breastfeeding. In the period between 6 weeks and 6 months, the EP should be used with caution, only if there are no alternatives, because the risks could outweigh the benefits, while after 6 months after childbirth, there are no problems with its use, provided that there are no other conditions that contraindicate its use.

Breastfeeding women should be informed that the evidence regarding the effects of taking combined oral contraceptives (COCs) on lactation and offspring is uncertain. However, the best-quality studies have shown no adverse effects of early estroprogestin intake on either successful breastfeeding (duration, exclusivity, initiation of complementary feeding) or infant outcomes (growth, health, and development) [25].

9.5.2 Progestogen-Only Contraception (POC)

Puerperium represents a great moment of vulnerability due to the neuroendocrine readjustment woman undergoes. Safe contraception can give the patient the stability she needs in terms of both prevention of VTE and mood disorders. A systematic review by Ti and Curtis, for example, reports that the use of POP, LNG-IUS, or medicated subcutaneous implant is associated with a 50% reduction in mood fluctuations and depressive state compared with COC, with which there is minimal worsening of these conditions [26]. Regarding migraine (both with and without aura), whose increase is due to oxytocin activating the trigeminal nerve, POP is the only hormonal contraception that can be prescribed, because it is not associated with increased risk of VTE, which is already higher in patients with migraine [27].

There are several types of progestogen-only contraception:

- Levonorgestrel or etonogestrel subcutaneous implant can be safely inserted at any time after delivery, as the advantages generally outweigh the theoretical or proven risks [24].
- Injectable methods: Although progestogen-only contraception has no apparent direct impact on breastfeeding and child health or development, the WHO still expresses theoretical concern about the potential exposure of the neonate to depo-medroxyprogesterone acetate (DMPA) and norethisterone enanthate and recommends delaying initiation of these methods until after 6 weeks postpartum [28].
- LNG—intrauterine system.
- Progestin-only pill (POP):
  Available data in literature confirm that the use of POPs does not adversely affect either the quantity and quality of breast milk or the child health and development. Therefore, this formulation, characterized by a good safety profile, can be proposed as the first choice of contraception both in the postpartum period and in the subsequent medium-long term. One of the most important problems that is typically found in POPs and that negatively affects adherence to treatment is the bleeding profile, which leads the patient to discontinue the therapy for frequent spotting. In this sense, drospirenone (DRSP) is the progestin that is associated with fewer episodes of unscheduled bleeding. The Food and Drug Administration evaluating the rate of withdrawal from therapy due to menstrual irregularity reports that only 4% of patients using DRPS abandoned their therapy. This molecule also has no negative impact on weight; it can be administered in women who are obese, smokers, older than 35 years of age, and with hypertension (also on antihypertensive treatment). DRSP is a safe choice for breastfeeding women

and for women who have a high VTE risk after pregnancy. The study by Melka et al. on the dosing concentration of DRSP in breast milk for 7 consecutive days in women with breastfeeding shows that the amount of DRSP that passes into 800 mL of breast milk 24 h after pill assumption is on average 4487 ng, which represents 0.11% of the daily dose (therefore absolutely unlikely to cause adverse effects in the newborn) [29]. DRSP does not cause problems of vaginal dryness or reduced bone mineral density in young patients, because unlike, for example, MPA, it does not decrease plasma circulating estrogen levels below 20–30 mg.

9.6   Conclusions

Fertility returns within 1 month of the end of pregnancy unless breastfeeding occurs. Breastfeeding, which itself suppresses fertility after childbirth, influences both when contraception should start and what methods can be used. Moreover, as numerous studies assert, short interpregnancy intervals appear to be associated with increased risks for adverse pregnancy outcomes for women of all ages. Maternal risks at short intervals may be greater for older women, whereas fetal and infant risks may be greater for younger women. In this scenery, a good counselling after delivery is mandatory in order to start contraception as soon as possible if adverse pregnancy outcomes are to be avoided.

References

1. World Health Organization (WHO) Programming strategies for postpartum family planning [Report]. Geneva: [s.n.]; 2013.
2. Schummers L, et al. Association of short interpregnancy interval with pregnancy outcomes according to maternal age [Article] // JAMA Intern Med. 2018.
3. Smith GCS, et al. Interpregnancy interval and risk of preterm birth and neonatal death: retrospective cohort study [Article] // BMJ. 2003.
4. Makins A, Cameron S. Post pregnancy contraception [Article] // Best Pract Res Clin Obstet Gynaecol. 2020.
5. Cleland J, et al. Family planning, contraception and health [Article] // The Lancet. 2012.
6. Ross JA, Winfrey WL. Contraceptive use, intention to use and unmet need during the extended postpartum period [Article] // International family planning perspectives. 2001.
7. RCOG Contraception after pregnancy [Article] // Faculty of Sexual and Reproductive Healthcare of the Royal College of the Obstetricians and Gynaecologists (FSRH). London: [s.n.]; 2017.
8. FFPRHC Guidance Contraceptive choices for breastfeeding women [Article] // J Fam Plann Reprod Health Care. 2004.
9. Glazier A, Mc Neilly AS, Howie PW. Hormonal background of lactational infertility [Article] // Int J Fertil. 1988.
10. Labbok MH, et al. Multicenter study of the Lactational Amenorrhea Method (LAM): I. Efficacy, duration, and implications for clinical application [Article] // Contraception. 1997.
11. Van der Wijden C, Manion C. Lactational amenorrhoea method for family planning [Article] // Cochrane Database Syst Rev. 2015.
12. Van der Wijden C, Brown J, Kleijnen J. Lactational amenorrhea for family planning [Article] // Cochrane database Syst Rev. 2008.

13. Mc Neilly AS, et al. Fertility after childbirth: adequacy of post-partum luteal phases [Article] // Clin Endocrinol. 1982.
14. Envision Sexual and Reproductive Health. PATH questions. [Report]. 2018.
15. Dehlendorf C, et al. Shared decision making in contraceptive counseling. [Article] // Contraception. 2017.
16. World Health Organization Medical eligibility criteria for contraceptive use [Article]. 2009.
17. Glasier A, et al. Contraception after pregnancy [Article] // Acta Obstet Gynecol Scand. 2019.
18. Labbock MH, et al. The Lactational Amenorrhea method (LAM): a post-partum introductory family planning method with policy and program implications [Article] // Advances in contraception. 1994.
19. Peterson AE, et al. Multicenter study of the Lactational Amenorrhea Method (LAM) III: effectiveness, duration, and satisfaction with reduced client provider contact [Article] // Contraception. 2000.
20. Hillis SD, et al. Poststerilization regret: findings from the United States Collaborative Review of sterilization [Article] // Obstet Gynecol. 1999.
21. Peterson HB, et al. The risk of pregnancy after tubal sterilization: findings of the U.S. Collaborative Review of Sterilization [Article] // Am J Obstet Gynecol. 1996.
22. World Health Organization (WHO) Selective practice recommendation for contraceptive use [Article]. 2002.
23. Jatlaoui TC, et al. Intrauterine Device expulsion after postpartum placement: a systematic review and meta-analysis [Article] // Obstet Gynecol. 2018.
24. Curtis KM, et al. U.S. medical eligibility criteria for contraceptive use [Article] // MMWR Recomm Rep. 2016.
25. Lopez LM, et al. Combined hormonal versus nonhormonal versus progestin-only contraception in lactation. [Article] // Cochrane Database Syst Rev. 2015.
26. Ti A, Curits KM. Postpartum hormonal contraception use and incidence of postpartum depression: a systematic review [Article] // Eur J Contracept Reprod Health Care. 2019.
27. Nappi RE, et al. Hormonal contraception in women with migraine: is progestogen-only contraception a better choice? [Article] // J Headache Pain. 2013.
28. Phillips SJ, et al. Progestogen-only contraceptive use among breastfeeding women: a systematic review [Article] // Contraception. 2016.
29. Melka D, et al. A single-arm study to evaluate the transfer of drospirenone to breast milk after reaching steady state, following oral administration of 4 mg drospirenone in healthy lactating female volunteers [Article] // Women's Health. 2020:[s.n.].

Amenorrhea in Oncological Patients

10

Marta Caretto and Tommaso Simoncini

10.1 Introduction

Cancer is an important cause of morbidity and mortality worldwide, with 18.1 million new cases and 9.6 million cancer deaths worldwide in 2018 [1]. Breast cancer is the most common female cancer worldwide, followed by colorectal cancer in high-income countries and cervical cancer in low- and middle-income countries.

Worldwide, there were about 2.1 million newly diagnosed female breast cancer cases in 2018, accounting for almost one in four cancer cases among women. Approximately 20% of new breast cancer diagnoses occur in women under the age of 45, with almost all requiring chemotherapy and adjuvant endocrine therapy. With earlier detection and improved treatments, particularly in high-income countries, women are living longer after a cancer diagnosis [2].

At the time of diagnosis, a significant proportion of young patients are concerned about the possible impact of anticancer treatments on their fertility and future chances of conception. Considering the rising trend in delaying childbearing and the higher number of patients who have not completed their family planning at the time of diagnosis, the demand for fertility preservation and information about the feasibility and safety of pregnancy following treatment completion is expected to increase [3].

One of the main issues that influence patients' quality of life after adjuvant chemotherapy is the risk for infertility [4]. Chemotherapy-induced amenorrhea (CIA) is a well-known toxicity after chemotherapy in young cancer patients that has been traditionally referred to as a marker of infertility. The majority of young cancer patients have concerns about treatment-induced infertility, and in some cases, these concerns

M. Caretto · T. Simoncini (✉)
Division of Obstetrics and Gynecology, Department of Clinical and Experimental Medicine,
University of Pisa, Pisa, Italy
e-mail: tommaso.simoncini@med.unipi.it

© International Society of Gynecological Endocrinology 2023
A. R. Genazzani et al. (eds.), *Amenorrhea*, ISGE Series,
https://doi.org/10.1007/978-3-031-22378-5_10

influence their treatment decision [5–8]. However, the discussion about CIA and infertility risk between oncologists and their patients remains limited [5, 6]. The link between adjuvant chemotherapy and amenorrhea has been well established, but the specific effect of individual chemotherapeutic agents and regimens on the risk for amenorrhea has not been well characterized. The most important drawback on the current literature is the lack of uniform definition of CIA. In the mid-1990s, a systematic review by Bines et al. underscored the need for uniform definition of CIA and proposed one based on the duration of amenorrhea (>6 months) [9]. A similar definition has been adopted from the American College of Obstetricians and Gynecologists based on the current systematic review and the evidence derived from studies with long-term follow-up, where resumption of menses occurs often within 2 years of CIA [10, 11]; Zavos and Valachis suggested that the definition of CIA should be based on the presence of amenorrhea for at least 2 years commencing within 2 years of chemotherapy with no resumption of menses during this period. One could argue that this definition is also problematic since there are some patients that resume menses even 2–3 years after CIA [12]; however, they assumed that the 2-year cutoff is an acceptable compromise between the necessity for a uniform and reliable definition and the resources that a prospective study investigating the risk for CIA in cancer patients needs.

Irrespective of the definition used for CIA, cessation of menses is only a surrogate marker for ovarian function and should not be considered synonymous to true ovarian failure. In fact, it has been found that estrogen levels can remain high despite the presence of CIA for more than 12 months [12]. Conversely, recovery of menstruation after chemotherapy does not rule out follicular depletion and fertility cannot be guaranteed [13]. These observations suggest that more accurate indicators of ovarian function are needed to properly inform cancer patients about their risk for infertility due to cancer treatment. Among several markers that have been studied, anti-Müllerian hormone (AMH) seems to be the most promising one. Indeed, serum AMH has been associated with the recovery of ovarian function in young women during and after chemotherapy [14].

10.2 Etiologies and Pathogenesis

10.2.1 Gonadotoxicity of Anticancer Treatments

Cancer and anticancer treatments may affect posttreatment ovarian function by a reduction in ovarian reserve (i.e., the primordial follicle pool); a disturbed hormonal balance; or anatomical or functional changes to the ovaries, uterus, cervix, or vagina. Reduced ovarian function may result in infertility and premature ovarian insufficiency (POI): POI is defined as oligo/amenorrhea for >4 months and follicle-stimulating hormone (FSH) levels of >25 IU/L on two occasions, 4 weeks apart, before the age of 40 years. Notably, in cancer patients, menstrual function can resume many months after completion of treatment; in addition, infertility and POI may occur despite temporary resumption of menses [3].

   CIA is mainly due to damage to growing follicles that occurs within weeks after CIA initiation and is often transient. Depending on age, pretreatment ovarian reserve, and type of treatment, exhaustion of the primordial follicle pool may occur with subsequent POI. Because of their cell cycle-nonspecific mode of action, alkylating agents induce the greatest damage, not only to growing follicles but also to oocytes, resulting in a striking reduction of the primordial follicle pool [15].

   The impact of most targeted agents (including monoclonal antibodies and small molecules) and immunotherapy is largely unknown. Limited data for the antihuman epidermal growth factor receptor 2 (HER2) agents trastuzumab and/or lapatinib indicate no apparent gonadotoxicity [16]. An increased risk of ovarian dysfunction in patients treated with bevacizumab cannot be excluded [3]. Endocrine treatments may have an indirect effect on fertility by delaying time to pregnancy. A higher risk of treatment-related amenorrhea with the use of tamoxifen following chemotherapy has been described in several studies. Nonetheless, no impact on AMH levels has been shown [17, 18].

10.3   Prognostic Factors

Women who have had cancer are at an increased risk of early menopause and POI as a result of ovarian follicle depletion, stromal fibrosis, and vascular injury after chemotherapy and radiotherapy [19]. Early menopause has a negative effect on the quality of life [20] and is associated with osteoporosis, cardiovascular disease, and psychosocial disorders such as depression. Even survivors in whom ovarian function resumes or is maintained after cancer treatment might face a shortened *window of fertility* [21]. The extent of damage to the ovary depends on the type and dose of chemotherapy [3], radiotherapy dose, fractionation scheme, irradiation field [22], and the ovarian reserve before treatment (Table 10.1).

   Regarding the risk factors for CIA, age is the strongest risk factor (sixfold increased risk for CIA for patients <40 years old), whereas tamoxifen use is associated with nearly twofold increased risk for CIA. On the contrary, age at menarche and BMI do not influence the risk for CIA. These observations are supported by high level of evidence [12]. Age is an important marker of ovarian reserve, as are the serum markers estradiol, inhibin B, follicle-stimulating hormone, and AMH. AMH has emerged as an especially strong predictor of ovarian function after chemotherapy. A rapid and substantial reduction of circulating AMH concentrations is noted in adults after the start of chemotherapy [23], and recent data suggest that AMH concentrations before the start of chemotherapy, and the reduction and recovery of AMH during and after chemotherapy, might predict the amount of ovarian damage [24]. These data suggest a crucial role for AMH in the identification of patients who might benefit from fertility preservation and the approach that will optimize future fecundity. However, in prepubertal and peripubertal girls, AMH concentrations should be interpreted with caution because they cannot unequivocally predict reproductive life span [21]. Long-term follow-up data for AMH concentrations decades after cancer treatment are not yet available to establish the predictive potential of AMH with regard to reproductive life span in cancer survivors.

Table 10.1 Risks of treatment-related amenorrhea in female patients[a]

Degree of risk	Treatment type/regimen	Comments
High risk (>80%)[b]	Hematopoietic stem cell transplantation (especially alkylating agent-based myeloablative conditioning with cyclophosphamide, busulfan, melphalan, or total-body RT)	
	EBRT >6 Gy to a field including the ovaries	
	6 cycles of CMF, CEF, CAF, or TAC in women of >40 years	Significant decline in AMH levels after treatment, early menopause
	6e8 cycles of escalated BEACOPP in women of >30 years	Significant decline in AMH levels after treatment
Intermediate risk (20–80%)[c]	6 cycles of CMF, CEF, CAF, or TAC in women of 30–39 years	Significant decline in AMH levels after treatment, early menopause
	4 cycles of AC in women of >40 years	Significant decline in AMH levels after treatment
	4 cycles of AC/EC/taxane	Significant decline in AMH levels after treatment
	4 cycles of dd (F)EC/dd taxane	
	6e8 cycles of escalated BEACOPP in women of <30 years	Significant decline in AMH levels after treatment
	6 cycles of CHOP in women of >35 years	Early menopause
	6 cycles of DA-EPOCH in women of >35 years	Significant decline in AMH levels after treatment
	FOLFOX in women of >40 years	
Low risk (<20%)[d]	6 cycles of CMF, CEF, CAF, or TAC in women of <30 years	Significant decline in AMH levels after treatment, early menopause
	4 cycles of AC in women of <40 years	Significant decline in AMH levels after treatment
	2 cycles of escalated BEACOPP	Significant decline in AMH levels after treatment
	ABVD	Insignificant decline in AMH levels after treatment
	6 cycles of CHOP in women of <35 years	Early menopause
	6 cycles of DA-EPOCH in women of <35 years	Significant decline in AMH levels after treatment
	AML therapy (anthracycline/cytarabine)	Insignificant decline in AMH levels after treatment
	ALL therapy (multi-agent)	Insignificant decline in AMH levels after treatment
	Multi-agent ChT for osteosarcoma (doxorubicin, cisplatin, methotrexate, ifosfamide) in women of <35 years	

Table 10.1 (continued)

Degree of risk	Treatment type/regimen	Comments
	Multi-agent ChT for Ewing's sarcoma (doxorubicin, vincristine, dactinomycin, cyclophosphamide, ifosfamide, etoposide) in women of <35 years	
	FOLFOX in women of >40 years	
	Antimetabolites and vinca alkaloids	
	BEP or EP in women of <30 years	
	Radioactive iodine (I-131)	Decline in AMH levels after treatment
	Bevacizumab	
Unknown risk	Platinum- and taxane-based ChT	
	Most targeted therapies (including monoclonal antibodies and small molecules)	
	Immunotherapy	

ABVD doxorubicin, bleomycin, vinblastine, dacarbazine, *AC* doxorubicin, cyclophosphamide, *ALL* acute lymphoid leukemia, *AMH* anti-Müllerian hormone, *AML* acute myeloid leukemia, *BEACOPP* bleomycin, etoposide, doxorubicin, cyclophosphamide, vincristine, prednisone, procarbazine, *BEP* bleomycin, etoposide, cisplatin, *CAF* cyclophosphamide, doxorubicin, 5-fluorouracil, *CEF* cyclophosphamide, epirubicin, 5-fluorouracil, *CHOP* cyclophosphamide, doxorubicin, vincristine, prednisone, *ChT* chemotherapy, *CMF* cyclophosphamide, methotrexate, 5-fluorouracil, *DA-EPOCH* dose-adjusted etoposide, prednisone, vincristine, cyclophosphamide, doxorubicin, *dd* dose dense, *EBRT* external beam radiotherapy, *EC* epirubicin, cyclophosphamide, *EP* etoposide, cisplatin, *F* fluorouracil, *FOLFOX* folinic acid, 5-fluorouracil, oxaliplatin, *Gy* Gray, *RT* radiotherapy, *TAC* docetaxel, doxorubicin, cyclophosphamide
[a] Adapted from [3]
[b] >80% risk of permanent amenorrhea
[c] >40–60% risk of permanent amenorrhea
[d] <20% risk of permanent amenorrhea

Follicle depletion is the hallmark of ovarian damage and is most pronounced in women given alkylating agents, such as cyclophosphamide, [24] and in those who receive total-body irradiation before hemopoietic stem cell transplantation or direct irradiation of the ovaries. The precise mechanism by which cyclophosphamide affects the primordial follicle pool is not entirely understood, but recent studies investigating the effect of cyclophosphamide in mouse ovaries suggest that cyclophosphamide results in activation rather than apoptosis of primordial follicles [25], via upregulation of the PI3K/PTEN/Akt signaling pathway. According to these data, cyclophosphamide causes apoptosis of larger growing follicles, with cyclophosphamide-induced primordial follicle activation ultimately resulting in follicle burnout.

Other chemotherapeutic drugs might directly damage the growing oocyte or the highly proliferative granulosa cells within the developing follicle. These drugs might also cause follicle depletion indirectly, by damaging growing follicles and enhancing recruitment of primordial follicles to deplete the follicle pool, or by altering the ovarian stroma [19]. An understanding of the gonadotoxic mechanisms of chemotherapy is needed to design effective agents that protect against iatrogenic depletion of ovarian follicles in young patients with cancer.

Taking into account the effect of fertility issues on patients' quality of life, the American Society of Clinical Oncology recommends that oncologists discuss the risk of infertility and fertility preservation options in patients with cancer as early as possible before treatment starts [12].

10.4 Chemotherapy-Induced Ovarian Failure

Chemotherapy-associated ovarian failure (COF) refers to the disruption of both endocrine and reproductive ovarian function, after exposure to chemotherapy. It is defined as either the absence of regular menses in premenopausal female patients or increased FSH levels (>40 IU/L) [26].

In 2006, the American Society of Clinical Oncology attempted to sort antineo-plastic regimens, according to the associated fertility compromise risk. Hematopoietic stem cell transplant (HSCT) initiation regimens steadily compromise patients' fertility, while gonadotoxicity of adjuvant chemotherapy regimens against early breast cancer varies with duration of exposure and patient's age. Characteristically, triple-agent combinations, such as CMF (cyclophosphamide, methotrexate, fluorouracil), entail a high risk of infertility if administered for more than four cycles in women older than 40, whereas the risk is significantly reduced for younger patients. Notably, vincristine, methotrexate, and fluorouracil do not impose considerable fertility hazards, while there are no sufficient data regarding taxanes, oxaliplatin, and targeted treatments [27].

Considering the finite number of follicles available in the ovaries and their coexistence in different stages of development, variable pathophysiologic mechanisms have been proposed to underlie chemotherapy-induced ovarian failure. These include the following:

– "Accelerated" ovarian follicle maturation: Chemotherapy agents induce apoptosis of mature, functioning ovarian follicles, resulting in depression of estrogen and anti-Müllerian hormone negative feedback on the gonadotropic cells of the anterior pituitary. Constantly elevated gonadotropins may accelerate maturation of premature ovarian follicles, which, in their turn, enter apoptosis under systematic chemotherapy, thus leading to the gradual exhaustion of ovarian follicle deposit [26, 28]. Supporting evidence comes from histology studies of murine ovarian tissue, in cyclophosphamide-treated mice, showing increased population of early-growing follicles, in parallel with elimination of the quiescent ones. The enhanced phosphorylation of proteins involved in the maturation of primordial follicles seems to be mediated via the PI3K/PTEN/Akt signaling pathway, which may also be activated due to a direct effect of chemotherapy on oocytes and on pregranulosa cells supporting them [25].

– Direct quiescent follicle DNA damage: Non-cell cycle-specific chemotherapeu-
  tics, such as alkylating agents and doxorubicin, can induce the formation of cross-
  links in the DNA of nondividing, dormant oocytes. The subsequent accumulation
  of DNA strand breaks activates the pro-apoptotic intracellular pathways, leading to
  apoptosis of the affected ovarian follicles [29]. Relevant supporting evidence
  derives from studies of human oocyte in vitro cultures and human ovarian xenograft murine models, exposed to doxorubicin and cyclophosphamide, revealing
  double-strand breaks and features of apoptotic death in premature oocytes [27].
– Disrupted ovarian vascularization: Chemotherapy may compromise the functionality of ovarian vasculature and stroma supporting the gonadal cells. Local
  vascular spasm reducing ovarian blood flow, fibrosis of the ovarian cortex affecting blood vessel formation, and inhibition of angiogenesis are some of the
  described associated mechanisms. Relative evidence has been found in in vitro
  and murine xenograft studies of human ovarian tissue, as well as mouse ovaries,
  exposed to doxorubicin [27, 29].

10.5   Radiotherapy-Induced Ovarian Failure

Radiotherapy (RT) exposure causes a reduction in the number of ovarian follicles
and has an adverse effect on uterine and endometrial function; the gonadotoxic
effect of RT is dependent on the RT field, dose, and fractionation schedule, with
single doses more toxic than multiple fractions [3]. RT-related ovarian follicle loss
already occurs at doses higher than 2 Gy. The effective sterilizing dose at which
97.5% of patients are expected to develop immediate POI decreases with increasing
age at the time of treatment, ranging from 16 Gy at 20 years to 14 Gy at 30 years.
RT also induces loss of uterine elasticity in a dose-dependent manner. This inter-
feres with uterine distension, with increased risk throughout pregnancy [30]. A
potential negative impact of cancer on ovarian reserve has been described for young
women with lymphoma but not for patients with other malignancies.

10.5.1   Predicting Age of Ovarian Failure After Radiation

As survival rates for children and adolescents treated for cancer continue to improve,
a population of young women of reproductive age emerges for whom issues of fertile potential are paramount. Impaired fecundity and premature ovarian failure are
recognized potential late sequelae of radiotherapy to the ovaries [22].
   The human ovary contains a fixed pool of primordial oocytes, maximal at
5 months of gestational age, which declines with increasing age in a biexponential
fashion, culminating in the menopause at an average age of 50–51 years. For any
given age, the size of the oocyte pool can be estimated based on a mathematical
model of decline [22, 31]. The rate of oocyte decline represents an instantaneous
rate of temporal change determined by the remaining population pool, which
increases around age 37 years when approximately 25,000 primordial oocytes

remain and precedes the menopause by 12–14 years [32]. Reproductive aging in women is due to ovarian oocyte depletion with approximately 1000 oocytes remaining at the menopause. Assessment of ovarian reserve and reproductive age in healthy women remains a challenge.

Radiotherapy may be used either alone or in combination with surgery and chemotherapy to provide local disease control for solid tumors. Because of its established late sequelae on immature and developing tissues, irradiation is used cautiously, especially in children and adolescents. Total body, craniospinal axis, whole abdominal, or pelvic irradiation potentially exposes the ovaries to irradiation and may cause premature ovarian failure. The degree of impairment is related to the volume treated, total radiation dose, fractionation schedule, and age at the time of treatment [31, 33]. The number of primordial oocytes present at the time of treatment, together with the biologic dose of radiotherapy received by the ovaries, will determine the fertile "window" and influence the age at premature ovarian failure. Assessing the extent of radiation-induced damage of the primordial oocytes and predicting the impact on fertile potential have been challenging. An understanding of ovarian follicle dynamics has allowed us to determine the radiosensitivity of the human oocyte to be 2 Gy [33]. Application of this estimate has made it possible to determine the surviving fraction of the primordial oocyte pool for a given dose of radiotherapy and therefore predict the age (with confidence intervals) of premature ovarian failure by applying a mathematical model of decay.

Radiotherapy is frequently used in combination with chemotherapy for the treatment of cancer. Potentially, gonadotoxic chemotherapy may be a contributory factor to the development of a premature menopause. However, when the dose of radiotherapy received by the ovaries is at, or approaching, the effective sterilizing dose, the additional contribution of chemotherapy is likely to be minimal. For smaller doses of radiation to the ovary, such as for spinal irradiation, the contribution of chemotherapy will play a more significant role. Several agents have been described to cause ovarian damage, including procarbazine, chlorambucil, and cyclophosphamide with the extent of damage dependent on the agent administered and dose received [22]. As with radiotherapy, progressively smaller doses are required to produce ovarian failure with increasing age, reflecting the natural decline in the oocyte pool. Although the mechanism of cytotoxic chemotherapy-induced damage to the ovary is uncertain, exhaustion of the oocyte pool is likely.

A successful term pregnancy will depend on a normally functioning hypothalamic-pituitary-ovarian axis and a uterine environment that is not only receptive to implantation but also able to accommodate normal growth of the fetus. The degree of damage to the uterus depends on the total radiation dose and the site of irradiation. The prepubertal uterus is more vulnerable to the effects of pelvic irradiation with doses of radiation between 14 and 30 Gy likely to result in uterine dysfunction. High-dose pelvic radiotherapy in young women will have long-term effects on the uterine vasculature and development.

When counseling patients after treatment with smaller doses of radiotherapy, around 3 Gy, which can be associated with radiotherapy to the craniospinal axis, the physicians could be relatively optimistic and reassuring that they will have a significant reproductive window before premature ovarian failure occurs. The fertile window will be attenuated with increasing doses of radiotherapy. For girls who are likely to be rendered sterile before the onset of menarche, it will enable physicians to realistically counsel their patients and families when discussing options for preservation of ovarian function at the time of diagnosis before treatment has commenced. A number of strategies to protect the ovaries and preserve fertility during cancer therapy have been attempted [21, 34]. Limitation of radiation dose to the ovary is sometimes practiced in adult women, but in children it is technically difficult.

10.6   Prophylactic Menstrual Suppression

CIA is not the only situation of menstrual absence: Obstetrician–gynecologists are frequently consulted either before the initiation of cancer treatment to request menstrual suppression or during an episode of severe heavy bleeding to stop bleeding emergently.

Adolescents undergoing cancer treatment are at high risk of abnormal menstrual bleeding as a direct result of hematologic malignancies or as a secondary effect of chemotherapy, radiation therapy, or pretreatment regimens for stem cell or bone marrow transplantation, all of which may induce myelosuppression leading to thrombocytopenia. Additional considerations include the potential for disruption of the hypothalamic–pituitary–gonadal axis during cancer treatment leading to anovulatory bleeding. Also, even normal menstrual blood loss may pose a threat to adolescents who already are anemic, thrombocytopenic, or both, from hematologic malignancies or cancer treatments. Thus, obstetrician–gynecologists are frequently consulted either before the initiation of cancer treatment to request menstrual suppression or during an episode of severe heavy bleeding to stop bleeding emergently [35]. Therapy for both menstrual suppression and management of acute bleeding episodes should be tailored to the patient, the cancer diagnosis and treatment plan, and the individual's contraceptive needs. Because of the complex nature of cancer care, collaboration with the adolescent's oncologist is highly recommended. Options for menstrual suppression include gonadotropin-releasing hormone agonist (GnRHa), progestin-only therapy, and combined hormonal contraception [36]. Adolescents presenting emergently with severe uterine bleeding usually require only medical management; surgical management is rarely required. Considerations when choosing an appropriate treatment for acute bleeding include the patient's current menstrual status, current hemoglobin and platelet count, expected nadirs, planned cancer treatments, risk of thromboembolism, and request for contraception. If a patient is treated with leuprolide acetate for menstrual suppression, this should not be considered a contraceptive method because ovulation may not be universally suppressed [37].

An American College of Obstetricians and Gynecologists' Committee on Adolescent Health Care has been updated to make treatment recommendations based on more recent studies, to address specific concerns about the use of combined hormonal contraception (CHC) in cancer patients, and to update nonmedical management to include the intrauterine Foley balloon.

10.7 Menstrual Suppression

10.7.1 Gonadotropin-Releasing Hormone Agonists

Gonadotropin-releasing hormone agonists are highly effective at inducing menstrual suppression when initiated before cancer treatment [36]. The primary role of GnRHa is for menstrual suppression. Though they appear to have a protective effect on the ovary during chemotherapy in terms of resumption of menstruation and treatment-related premature ovarian failure, there is no conclusive evidence demonstrating the efficacy of GnRHa in fertility preservation [37].

Most of the data on GnRHa focuses on the use of leuprolide acetate, a synthetic GnRHa that acts as a potent inhibitor of gonadotropin release when given in therapeutic doses. Studies, including a systematic review of women undergoing cancer treatment, report high rates of amenorrhea with leuprolide acetate (ranging from 73 to 96%) [38].

After an initial flare response that causes a transient increase in circulating gonadotropins and sex steroids, leuprolide acetate reliably causes a hypoestrogenic state in 2 weeks. Therefore, bleeding may occur for 2–3 weeks after the first injection until hormone levels decrease and endometrial proliferation ceases. When initiating treatment with leuprolide, adding norethindrone acetate 5 mg daily will help mitigate breakthrough bleeding and other adverse effects of leuprolide. It may be given in doses of 3.75 mg intramuscularly monthly or 11.5 mg intramuscularly every 12 weeks. The 12-week formulation decreases the risk of more frequent monthly injections that may be due at a time of treatment-induced thrombocytopenia. If intramuscular injections are contraindicated, subcutaneous formulations are available [37].

Disadvantages of leuprolide acetate include the expected adverse effects related to a low-estrogen state, such as vasomotor symptoms and bone density loss. When leuprolide acetate is used to treat endometriosis in adolescents, add-back therapy with a progestin (such as norethindrone acetate 5 mg once daily) has been shown to preserve bone mass and substantially reduce vasomotor symptoms without increasing the rate of bleeding. Treatment should be individualized; certain cancer patients, depending on the potential risks and benefits, may be candidates for combined add-back therapy.

10.7.2 Progestin-Only Therapy

Daily administration of oral progestins allows for decreased endometrial proliferation and prevention of menses. Options for progestin-only oral therapies are medroxyprogesterone acetate (10–20 mg/day), norethindrone acetate (5–15 mg/day), drospirenone (4 mg/day), and norethindrone (0.35 mg/day). Drospirenone (4 mg/day) and norethindrone (0.35 mg/day) also provide contraception but do not confer the same degree of amenorrhea as other oral progestins, and unscheduled bleeding is relatively common in users [38, 39].

Use of depot medroxyprogesterone acetate (DMPA) results in relatively high rates of amenorrhea over time, with rates at 12–24 months reaching approximately

50–70% in the general population [40]. However, initial irregular bleeding with DMPA makes it a less reliable method for rapid therapeutic menstrual suppression and episodes of breakthrough bleeding can be challenging to manage, particularly in patients who are not candidates for adjuvant estrogen. It is classified as a Category 2 method (the advantages of using the method generally outweigh the theoretical or proven risks) among those with a history of VTE and active cancer according to the Centers for Disease Control and Prevention's U.S. Medical Eligibility Criteria for Contraceptive Use. Data on the use of progestin-only methods by patients with cancer are limited. Depot medroxyprogesterone acetate typically is administered every 12 weeks, but the dosing interval can be shortened to achieve amenorrhea quickly. Its long dosing interval of up to 3 months minimizes concerns over adherence and is a good option for patients unable to swallow or tolerate pills. A subcutaneous formulation (dose of 104 mg) is available and is recommended for adolescents with thrombocytopenia who are at risk of developing an intramuscular hematoma with intramuscular administration [37].

Although there are limited data regarding menstrual management with an LNG-IUD in patients undergoing cancer treatment, it is a reasonable option to manage heavy menstrual bleeding in a patient with benign or malignant disease. Furthermore, the World Health Organization and the Centers for Disease Control and Prevention state that IUDs can be used safely in women with immunosuppression because of cancer treatment. Although initial irregular bleeding may limit its use, many studies in noncancer patients have demonstrated the superiority of the 52 µg LNG-IUD over oral medroxyprogesterone acetate, norethindrone acetate, DMPA, and CHC for long-term menstrual control [37].

If an adolescent had an LNG-IUD or the etonogestrel single-rod implant inserted before her cancer diagnosis and has infrequent bleeding or amenorrhea, it is reasonable to continue the method for menstrual suppression. However, if an adolescent had an implant inserted before her cancer diagnosis and experiences bothersome bleeding, the bleeding can be temporized with a norethindrone acetate or medroxyprogesterone taper and the implant continued.

10.7.3 Combined Hormonal Contraceptives

When used continuously, CHCs are effective for producing amenorrhea, although complete amenorrhea cannot be guaranteed. The Centers for Disease Control and Prevention's 2016 U.S. Medical Eligibility Criteria for Contraceptive Use notes that when oral contraceptives are primarily used as therapy, rather than to prevent pregnancy, even in women where contraceptive use might be cautioned against or contraindicated (such as in those with cancer), the benefits from therapeutic use might outweigh the risks [37].

The decision to use estrogen in patients with cancer should be tailored to the individual patient after collaborative consideration of the risk–benefit ratio with the patient and the healthcare team; the patient should be closely monitored for known adverse effects such as liver toxicity and VTE.

10.7.4 Emergent Treatment of Acute Uterine Bleeding

Some adolescents may present with life-threatening bleeding in the setting of a new cancer diagnosis, whereas others who are undergoing myelosuppressive treatment may not have the time to benefit from prophylactic menstrual suppression and need more urgent therapy once bleeding occurs. Medical management is the initial approach for patients who are experiencing an episode of acute heavy bleeding. Surgical management should be considered for patients who are not clinically stable, or for those whose conditions are not suitable for medical management or who have failed to respond appropriately to medical management [41]. Some hormonal therapies that are used for menstrual suppression, such as leuprolide acetate, DMPA, LNG-IUD, and etonogestrel implant, are not appropriate for the initial management of acute heavy bleeding because the onset of action is delayed, and, in some cases, the bleeding pattern is unpredictable. Instead, these therapies may be used in conjunction with therapy for acute bleeding to prevent future episodes of acute uterine bleeding. Ultrasonography can be useful to guide management. Endometrial thickness can guide whether the patient may benefit from progestin or estrogen.

10.8 Fertility Preservation Strategies

The assessment of fertility risk and the selection of an individualized strategy to optimize fecundity after cancer treatment are huge challenges and require intense cooperation between fertility preservation specialists, oncologists, other healthcare workers, and the patient. Guidelines developed on the basis of systematic reviews and scientific literature analyses recommend fertility preservation approaches by patient age, cancer type, type of treatment, presence of a male partner or patient preference for the use of banked donor sperm, time available for fertility preservation intervention, and likelihood of ovarian metastasis. Established fertility preservation methods include oocyte and embryo cryopreservation, both derived from routine reproductive clinical practice, and ovarian transposition (oophoropexy), which can be offered to women undergoing pelvic irradiation [21] (Fig. 10.1).

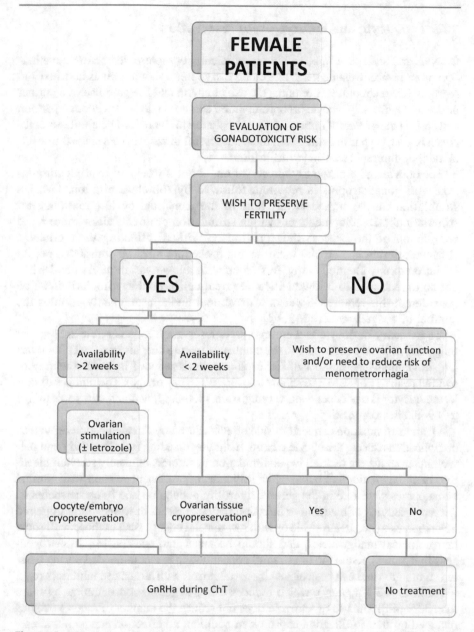

Fig. 10.1 Management flowchart for ovarian function and/or fertility preservation in female patients. *ChT* chemotherapy, *GnRHa* gonadotropin-releasing hormone agonist. [a]To be offered preferably in women 36 years of age and to be considered with particular caution in cases of acute leukemia, or any solid tumor or hematological disease with pelvic involvement. Adapted from [21]

10.8.1 Oocyte and Embryo Cryopreservation

Oocytes and embryos can be safely and efficiently cryopreserved before the initiation of anticancer treatments. While embryo cryopreservation is an established and reproducible technology, it requires the use of sperm and the presence of a partner or donor. Conversely, oocyte cryopreservation can be carried out without a partner, and so it is the preferred option for most postpubertal women. The ability to cryopreserve oocytes has become much more successful in recent years since the development of ultrarapid freezing (vitrification).

For oocyte and embryo cryopreservation, about 2 weeks of ovarian stimulation with gonadotropins is required, followed by follicle aspiration. Ovarian stimulation can be started at any time of the menstrual cycle ("random start stimulation"). Developments in ovarian stimulation protocols allow more rapid completion of the process than previously, without affecting their efficacy. However, timing is a crucial factor as the procedure must be completed before initiation of any chemotherapy. In women with a low ovarian reserve and without an urgent need to initiate anticancer treatments, double stimulation can be considered; this requires 4 weeks of treatment and approximately doubles the number of oocytes retrieved [3, 42].

The efficacy of oocyte and embryo cryopreservation to generate a subsequent pregnancy is tightly connected to the number of mature oocytes retrieved after ovarian stimulation. The number of retrieved oocytes is reduced in women with poor ovarian reserve (low AMH level due to ovarian surgery or age). The number of collected oocytes is age dependent, varying from 15.4–8.8 in women <26 years of age to 9.9–8.0 in women 36–40 years of age.

Ovarian stimulation can lead to side effects caused by the medication as well as complications during the oocyte pickup, including bleeding from the ovary and pelvic infection. Severe ovarian hyperstimulation syndrome, clinically relevant bleeding, or inflammation/infections after follicular aspiration in women with normal hematopoiesis are rare in the general infertility population and in cancer patients. An increased risk of bleeding or infection may be present in women with impaired hematopoiesis (i.e., neutropenic or with low platelet count), such as those with some hematological malignancies, and should be taken into account [3]. In estrogen-sensitive tumors, reduction of estradiol concentration is recommended during ovarian stimulation and can be achieved by co-treatment with aromatase inhibitors (e.g., letrozole 2×2.5 mg/day), which reduces estrogen serum concentration by more than 50% [43]. The use of letrozole does not reduce the number of mature oocytes obtained or their fertilization capacity; in addition, no effect on congenital abnormality rates in children has been observed.

Oocyte or embryo cryopreservation is indicated for women preferably <40 years of age who will be exposed to gonadotoxic anticancer therapies and who want to preserve their fertility. It is not indicated in women with serious coagulation defects or high risk of infections. Transabdominal monitoring and oocyte recovery may be possible in those for whom vaginal procedures are not possible or acceptable. Women choosing to store embryos created with their partner's sperm should be advised that the embryos will be the joint property of the couple; in the event of the relationship not continuing, there may be issues in using the embryos. An established collaboration between oncology and fertility units is crucial.

There is a need for data on all aspects of oocyte cryopreservation from larger series of women to clarify whether certain diagnoses may benefit from particular stimulation protocols, the effects on oocyte quality and most importantly cumulative live birth rates. Future studies are also needed to investigate the benefits of combining different fertility preservation methods to increase pregnancy rates.

10.8.2   Ovarian Tissue Cryopreservation

Ovarian tissue cryopreservation is an alternative approach for preserving fertility before gonadotoxic treatments. While it is still regarded as experimental in some countries, the American Society for Reproductive Medicine suggests that it should be considered as an established procedure to be offered to carefully selected patients [3, 44].

Biopsies of the ovarian cortex or unilateral ovariectomy are usually carried out by laparoscopy under general anesthesia. Although vitrification is quicker and less expensive, slow freezing remains the standard of care because almost all pregnancies achieved after transplantation have been obtained using this procedure. Ovarian tissue cryopreservation should be offered only in laboratories with specific expertise and facilities to support safe tissue cryopreservation and storage for subsequent autologous transplantation, with necessary regulation. The "hub and spoke" model, with ovarian surgery carried out locally and tissue transported to a central laboratory, may be preferred.

Transplantation, either orthotopic or heterotopic, is currently the only method available in clinical practice to restore ovarian function and fertility using cryopreserved ovarian tissue. As with oocyte and embryo cryopreservation, the main factor affecting success rate is age: women of younger age at ovarian tissue cryopreservation have better fertility outcomes after ovarian tissue transplantation than older women, with only a few pregnancies achieved in women over 36 years of age [45].

Ovarian tissue collection and transplantation are usually carried out by laparoscopy. Surgical risk is considered low, and complications (e.g., conversion laparotomy, bleeding, reintervention for cutaneous infection, bladder lesion, or minor complications) are rare (0.2–1.4%) [46]. The procedure should not be proposed to patients with high surgical/anesthesia risks related to their disease and ideally should be done at the same time as other procedures that require anesthesia. The risk of disease transmission during transplantation due to residual neoplastic cells within the ovarian cortex is one of the major safety concerns, especially in pelvic cancers or systemic diseases such as leukemia. Several diseases at advanced stages, such as Burkitt's lymphoma, non-Hodgkin's lymphoma, breast cancer, and sarcoma, might also carry a risk of ovarian involvement. Nevertheless, ovarian tissue should always be carefully analyzed before grafting using all available technologies, such as immunohistochemistry and molecular markers, according to the disease. Xenografting has also been used in this context. Data on children are reassuring as no congenital malformations have been reported [3].

Ovarian tissue cryopreservation is appropriate when the time available before starting anticancer treatments is too short for ovarian stimulation and oocyte or embryo cryopreservation. Although there is no clear consensus on the maximum age for ovarian tissue cryopreservation, it is usually recommended to offer this procedure only to women <36 years of age [3, 45]. Ovarian tissue cryopreservation can also be carried out after an initial, low-intensity gonadotoxic treatment regimen in order to reduce the risk of neoplastic cells being present in the ovary (i.e., in leukemia patients) or when the patient's initial health condition contraindicates an immediate procedure.

Research is ongoing to improve tissue function after grafting using several tools, including human adipose tissue-derived stem cells, mesenchymal stem cells, and decellularized scaffolds.

10.8.3   Ovarian Transposition and Gonadal Shielding During RT

Two options exist for protecting ovaries from RT: transposition of the ovaries before RT and gonadal shielding during RT.

Ovarian transposition outside the planned RT field is a routinely used technique to minimize ovarian follicle RT exposure. Although both laparotomic and laparoscopic approaches are possible, the procedure is mostly carried out by laparoscopy to accelerate recovery and avoid postponing RT [3]. The ovary is mobilized with its vascular pedicle, and the location is marked with radio-opaque clips to allow identification of the transposed ovary. It is possible to transpose only one ovary, but better results are achieved with a bilateral procedure. Transposition of the ovary into subcutaneous tissue is another option, but it is associated with a higher risk of cyst formation [47]. Transposed ovaries can be safely punctured for oocyte retrieval. In certain cases, ovaries can be returned to their original location after RT. The rate of retained ovarian function is approximately 65% in patients undergoing surgery and RT [48]. Reasons for failure include necrosis related to vascular impairment and migration after insufficient fixation. Success rate is influenced by the method of evaluation (presence of menstrual cycle, FSH levels, AMH levels) and the duration of follow-up (as ovarian function decreases over time). The surgical risk of ovarian transposition is similar to other gynecological procedures (i.e., risk of bowel and vessel injury). Risk of developing ovarian carcinoma in a transposed ovary is extremely low. This could be reduced even further when fallopian tubes are resected during the surgical procedure [48].

Gonadal shielding during RT by lead blocks reduces the expected RT dose to 4–5 Gy [3]. The minimum free margin should be 2 cm in order to reduce the risk of gonadal irradiation due to inner organ movement. Ovarian transposition and gonadal shielding are indicated in women <40 years of age who are scheduled to receive pelvic RT for cervical (if there is a low risk of ovarian metastasis or recurrence), vaginal, rectal, or anal cancers; Hodgkin's or non-Hodgkin's lymphoma in the pelvis; or Ewing's sarcoma of the pelvis. Long-term follow-up evaluating the risks of transposition and fertility rates after RT completion is needed.

10.8.4   Need to Reduce Gonadotoxicity: Medical Gonadoprotection

There has been extraordinary interest in medical agents that can potentially preserve fertility from the ovarian toxicity of chemotherapy. In this sense, temporary ovarian suppression obtained by administering a GnRHa has been studied as a strategy to reduce the gonadotoxic effect of chemotherapy [49]. When ovarian suppression with GnRHa is offered, GnRHa should be started at least 1 week before the initiation of systemic gonadotoxic treatment and prolonged until after the administration of the last chemotherapy cycle [50]. The debate on the efficacy of GnRHa for fertility preservation is still heated, but the 2018 ASCO guidelines recommended that GnRHa may be offered to premenopausal patients for reducing the likelihood of chemotherapy-induced ovarian insufficiency [51]. Nowadays, studies regarding the role of GnRHa as a fertility preservation treatment are evolving. In fact, the difference in the efficacy of GnRHa could not be assigned to the type of cancer, but rather to the regimen of chemotherapy. It is well known that gonadotoxic impact depends on the type of chemotherapeutic agent and the duration of administration [52]. The most common chemotherapy regimen used for the treatment of gynecological cancers (epithelial ovarian cancer) includes a combination of a platinum agent (carboplatin) and a taxane (paclitaxel). Currently, there is a lack of robust evidence to advise and recommend women on the risk of gonadotoxicity associated with this combination. Bleomycin, etoposide, and cisplatin (BEP)- or etoposide and cisplatin (EP)-chemotherapy regimens are often used for the treatment of non-epithelial ovarian cancers. Overall, chemotherapy regimens used for young women with gynecological cancers are considered to be associated with a low risk of gonadotoxicity, but this risk seems to be different according to the type of chemotherapy agent, the dose and length of exposure, and the age of the patient [3]. To investigate the impact of newer gonadotoxic treatments (including targeted agents and immunotherapy) on ovarian function, ovarian reserve and fertility potential of cancer patients should be considered a research priority. Instead, the gonadotoxic effect of chemotherapy in premenopausal women with early breast cancer is well known; the highest risk of gonadotoxicity is associated with the administration of the alkylating agent cyclophosphamide, commonly given as part of (neo)adjuvant chemotherapy regimens [53].

After more than 30 years of research and controversy in the gonadotoxicity battles, five theoretical mechanisms could explain how the GnRHa could minimize the gonadotoxic effect of chemotherapy:

1. Simulating the prepubertal hormonal milieu: GnRHa treatment has been identified to induce an initial release of gonadotropins, which desensitize the GnRH receptors on the pituitary gonadotropes, preventing pulsatile GnRH secretion, thus resulting in a hypogonadotropic, prepubertal hormonal milieu. In this prepubertal hypogonadotropic milieu, the follicles remain in the quiescent phase and are less vulnerable to chemotherapy-induced gonadotoxicity. Therefore, the administration of GnRHa, after the initial flare-up effect, decreases FSH concentration through pituitary desensitization, preventing the secretion of growth fac-

tors by the more advanced FSH-dependent follicles, and secondarily preserving more primordial follicles (PMFs), which are metabolically inactive, in the dormant stage.

2. Interrupting the burnout effect: The administration of GnRHa may interfere with the accelerated follicle recruitment induced by chemotherapy by desensitizing the GnRH receptors in the pituitary gland, preventing an increase of FSH level despite low estrogen and inhibin concentrations.

3. Decreased utero-ovarian perfusion: A result of the hypoestrogenic milieu generated by pituitary-gonadal desensitization. The decreased utero-ovarian perfusion could result in a reduction of exposure of the ovaries to chemotherapeutic agents' injuries.

4. A possible direct effect mediated by ovarian GnRH receptors: Human gonads also contain GnRH receptors, and the activation of the ovarian GnRH receptor may decrease apoptosis.

5. Possible protection of ovarian germinative stem cells (GSCs): In patients undergoing chemotherapy, high menopausal FSH levels and undetectable AMH levels have been observed. Approximately a year after the chemotherapeutic ovarian insult, FSH concentrations have been shown to decrease to normal levels and AMH has been found to increase in a large number of patients co-treated with GnRHa. Based on these clinical findings, it has been speculated that the administration of GnRHa may interact with these protected GSCs through some pathways essential for the initiation of folliculogenesis, maturation, and secretion of AMH, inhibin, and estrogens, and the latter two lead to a decrease in FSH levels to normal [54].

For premenopausal women interested in fertility preservation, with the hope of reducing chemotherapy-induced ovarian insufficiency and minimizing the gonadotoxic effect of treatments, temporary ovarian suppression with GnRHa during chemotherapy should not be considered an equivalent or alternative option for fertility preservation, but it should be proposed after embryo and oocyte cryopreservation. Temporary ovarian suppression during chemotherapy achieved by administering a GnRHa is the only strategy that has entered clinical use [55].

10.8.5 Life After Treatment

Although current oncofertility guidelines are universal among different tumor types and patient profiles, potential disparities between patients due to age, chemotherapy agents employed, and the malignancy itself may also interfere with fertility preservation practices. Consequently, a more methodical investigation of fertility preservation strategies, considering the above parameters, is required, in order to adequately establish the most efficient practices for each patient group.

At the time of diagnosis, a significant proportion of postpubertal patients have not completed their family planning and express a desire for pregnancy after treatment. Fertility depends on the female's stage in life (before or after puberty, before or after menopause), menstrual history, hormone levels, type of cancer and treatment, and treatment doses. Posttreatment pregnancy rates are highly dependent on the type of cancer, with the lowest rates reported for men with a history of acute leukemia or non-Hodgkin's lymphoma and for women with a history of breast or cervical cancer.

Because all these factors need to be considered, it can be hard to predict if a woman is likely to be fertile after chemotherapy. The feasibility and safety of using assisted reproductive technology (ART) following anticancer treatment are an important issue to be considered for adult cancer survivors who did not have access to fertility preservation strategies at the time of diagnosis and/or where there are difficulties with spontaneous conception. Female adult cancer survivors have a higher likelihood of undergoing fertility treatments compared with healthy women, with increasing use over time.

Funding   No external funding has been received for the preparation of this chapter.

Disclosure   No disclosure to declare.

References

1. Bray F, Ferlay J, Soerjomataram I, Siegel RL, Torre LA, Jemal A. Global cancer statistics 2018: GLOBOCAN estimates of incidence and mortality worldwide for 36 cancers in 185 countries. CA Cancer J Clin. 2018;68(6):394–424. https://doi.org/10.3322/caac.21492. Epub 2018 Sep 12.
2. Szabo RA, Marino JL, Hickey M. Managing menopausal symptoms after cancer. Climacteric. 2019;22:572. https://doi.org/10.1080/13697137.2019.1646718.
3. Lambertini M, Peccatori FA, Demeestere I, Amant F, Wyns C, Stukenborg JB, Paluch-Shimon S, Halaska MJ, Uzan C, Meissner J, von Wolff M, Anderson RA, Jordan K, ESMO Guidelines Committee, Electronic address: clinicalguidelines@esmo.org. Fertility preservation and post-treatment pregnancies in post-pubertal cancer patients: ESMO Clinical Practice Guidelines†. Ann Oncol. 2020;31(12):1664–78. https://doi.org/10.1016/j.annonc.2020.09.006. Epub 2020 Sep 22.
4. Howard-Anderson J, Ganz PA, Bower JE, Stanton AL. Quality of life, fertility concerns, and behavioral health outcomes in younger breast cancer survivors: a systematic review. J Natl Cancer Inst. 2012;104(5):386–405. https://doi.org/10.1093/jnci/djr541. Epub 2012 Jan 23.
5. Ruddy KJ, Gelber SI, Tamimi RM, Ginsburg ES, Schapira L, Come SE, Borges VF, Meyer ME, Partridge AH. Prospective study of fertility concerns and preservation strategies in young women with breast cancer. J Clin Oncol. 2014;32(11):1151–6. https://doi.org/10.1200/JCO.2013.52.8877. Epub 2014 Feb 24.
6. Partridge AH, Gelber S, Peppercorn J, Sampson E, Knudsen K, Laufer M, Rosenberg R, Przypyszny M, Rein A, Winer EP. Web-based survey of fertility issues in young women with breast cancer. J Clin Oncol. 2004;22(20):4174–83. https://doi.org/10.1200/JCO.2004.01.159. PMID: 15483028.
7. Llarena NC, Estevez SL, Tucker SL, Jeruss JS. Impact of fertility concerns on tamoxifen initiation and persistence. J Natl Cancer Inst. 2015;107(10):djv202. https://doi.org/10.1093/jnci/djv202. PMID: 26307641; PMCID: PMC5825683.

8. King JW, Davies MC, Roche N, Abraham JM, Jones AL. Fertility preservation in women undergoing treatment for breast cancer in the UK: a questionnaire study. Oncologist. 2012;17:910–6.

9. Bines J, Oleske DM, Cobleigh MA. Ovarian function in premenopausal women treated with adjuvant chemotherapy for breast cancer. J Clin Oncol. 1996;14(5):1718–29. https://doi.org/10.1200/JCO.1996.14.5.1718. PMID: 8622093.

10. Sukumvanich P, Case LD, Van Zee K, Singletary SE, Paskett ED, Petrek JA, Naftalis E, Naughton MJ. Incidence and time course of bleeding after long-term amenorrhea after breast cancer treatment: a prospective study. Cancer. 2010;116(13):3102–11. https://doi.org/10.1002/cncr.25106. PMID: 20564648.

11. Han HS, Ro J, Lee KS, Nam BH, Seo JA, Lee DH, Lee H, Lee ES, Kang HS, Kim SW. Analysis of chemotherapy-induced amenorrhea rates by three different anthracycline and taxane containing regimens for early breast cancer. Breast Cancer Res Treat. 2009;115(2):335–42. https://doi.org/10.1007/s10549-008-0071-9. Epub 2008 May 28. PMID: 18506620.

12. Zavos A, Valachis A. Risk of chemotherapy-induced amenorrhea in patients with breast cancer: a systematic review and meta-analysis. Acta Oncol. 2016;55(6):664–70. https://doi.org/10.3109/0284186X.2016.1155738. Epub 2016 Apr 22. PMID: 27105082.

13. Decanter C, Morschhauser F, Pigny P, Lefebvre C, Gallo C, Dewailly D. Anti-Mullerian hormone follow-up in young women treated by chemotherapy for lymphoma: preliminary results. Reprod Biomed Online. 2010;20:280–5.

14. Peigné M, Decanter C. Serum AMH level as a marker of acute and long-term effects of chemotherapy on the ovarian follicular content: a systematic review. Reprod Biol Endocrinol. 2014;12:26. https://doi.org/10.1186/1477-7827-12-26. PMID: 24666685; PMCID: PMC3987687.

15. Spears N, Lopes F, Stefansdottir A, Rossi V, De Felici M, Anderson RA, Klinger FG. Ovarian damage from chemotherapy and current approaches to its protection. Hum Reprod Update. 2019;25(6):673–93. https://doi.org/10.1093/humupd/dmz027. PMID: 31600388; PMCID: PMC6847836.

16. Lambertini M, Campbell C, Bines J, Korde LA, Izquierdo M, Fumagalli D, Del Mastro L, Ignatiadis M, Pritchard K, Wolff AC, Jackisch C, Lang I, Untch M, Smith I, Boyle F, Xu B, Barrios CH, Baselga J, Moreno-Aspitia A, Piccart M, Gelber RD, de Azambuja E. Adjuvant anti-HER2 therapy, treatment-related amenorrhea, and survival in premenopausal HER2-positive early breast cancer patients. J Natl Cancer Inst. 2019;111(1):86–94. https://doi.org/10.1093/jnci/djy094.

17. Zhao J, Liu J, Chen K, Li S, Wang Y, Yang Y, Deng H, Jia W, Rao N, Liu Q, Su F. What lies behind chemotherapy-induced amenorrhea for breast cancer patients: a meta-analysis. Breast Cancer Res Treat. 2014;145(1):113–28. https://doi.org/10.1007/s10549-014-2914-x. Epub 2014 Mar 27. PMID: 24671358.

18. Dezellus A, Barriere P, Campone M, Lemanski C, Vanlemmens L, Mignot L, Delozier T, Levy C, Bendavid C, Debled M, Bachelot T, Jouannaud C, Loustalot C, Mouret-Reynier MA, Gallais-Umbert A, Masson D, Freour T. Prospective evaluation of serum anti-Müllerian hormone dynamics in 250 women of reproductive age treated with chemotherapy for breast cancer. Eur J Cancer. 2017;79:72–80. https://doi.org/10.1016/j.ejca.2017.03.035. Epub 2017 Apr 29. PMID: 28463758.

19. Morgan S, Anderson RA, Gourley C, Wallace WH, Spears N. How do chemotherapeutic agents damage the ovary? Hum Reprod Update. 2012;18(5):525–35. https://doi.org/10.1093/humupd/dms022. Epub 2012 May 30.

20. Letourneau JM, Ebbel EE, Katz PP, Katz A, Ai WZ, Chien AJ, Melisko ME, Cedars MI, Rosen MP. Pretreatment fertility counseling and fertility preservation improve quality of life in reproductive age women with cancer. Cancer. 2012;118(6):1710–7. https://doi.org/10.1002/cncr.26459. Epub 2011 Sep 1.

21. De Vos M, Smitz J, Woodruff TK. Fertility preservation in women with cancer. Lancet. 2014;384(9950):1302–10. https://doi.org/10.1016/S0140-6736(14)60834-5. Erratum in: Lancet. 2015;385(9971):856. PMID: 25283571; PMCID: PMC4270060.

22. Wallace WH, Thomson AB, Saran F, Kelsey TW. Predicting age of ovarian failure after radiation to a field that includes the ovaries. Int J Radiat Oncol Biol Phys. 2005;62(3):738–44. https://doi.org/10.1016/j.ijrobp.2004.11.038. PMID: 15936554.

23. Decanter C, Morschhauser F, Pigny P, Lefebvre C, Gallo C, Dewailly D. Anti-Müllerian hormone follow-up in young women treated by chemotherapy for lymphoma: preliminary results. Reprod Biomed Online. 2010;20(2):280–5. https://doi.org/10.1016/j.rbmo.2009.11.010. Epub 2009 Dec 3.

24. Brougham MF, Crofton PM, Johnson EJ, Evans N, Anderson RA, Wallace WH. Anti-Müllerian hormone is a marker of gonadotoxicity in pre- and postpubertal girls treated for cancer: a prospective study. J Clin Endocrinol Metab. 2012;97(6):2059–67. https://doi.org/10.1210/jc.2011-3180. Epub 2012 Apr 3. PMID: 22472563.

25. Kalich-Philosoph L, Roness H, Carmely A, Fishel-Bartal M, Ligumsky H, Paglin S, Wolf I, Kanety H, Sredni B, Meirow D. Cyclophosphamide triggers follicle activation and "burnout"; AS101 prevents follicle loss and preserves fertility. Sci Transl Med. 2013;5(185):185ra62. https://doi.org/10.1126/scitranslmed.3005402. PMID: 23677591.

26. Cui W, Stern C, Hickey M, Goldblatt F, Anazodo A, Stevenson WS, Phillips KA. Preventing ovarian failure associated with chemotherapy. Med J Aust. 2018;209(9):412–6. https://doi.org/10.5694/mja18.00190. PMID: 30376664.

27. Mauri D, Gazouli I, Zarkavelis G, Papadaki A, Mavroeidis L, Gkoura S, Ntellas P, Amylidi AL, Tsali L, Kampletsas E. Chemotherapy associated ovarian failure. Front Endocrinol (Lausanne). 2020;11:572388. https://doi.org/10.3389/fendo.2020.572388. PMID: 33363515; PMCID: PMC7753213.

28. Roness H, Kashi O, Meirow D. Prevention of chemotherapy-induced ovarian damage. Fertil Steril. 2016;105(1):20–9. https://doi.org/10.1016/j.fertnstert.2015.11.043. Epub 2015 Dec 8. PMID: 26677788.

29. Bedoschi G, Navarro PA, Oktay K. Chemotherapy-induced damage to ovary: mechanisms and clinical impact. Future Oncol. 2016;12(20):2333–44. https://doi.org/10.2217/fon-2016-0176. Epub 2016 Jul 12. PMID: 27402553; PMCID: PMC5066134.

30. Brännström M, Dahm-Kähler P. Uterus transplantation and fertility preservation. Best Pract Res Clin Obstet Gynaecol. 2019;55:109–16. https://doi.org/10.1016/j.bpobgyn.2018.12.006. Epub 2018 Dec 21. PMID: 30711374.

31. Faddy MJ, Gosden RG. A model conforming the decline in follicle numbers to the age of menopause in women. Hum Reprod. 1996;11(7):1484–6. https://doi.org/10.1093/oxfordjournals.humrep.a019422. PMID: 8671489.

32. Richardson SJ, Senikas V, Nelson JF. Follicular depletion during the menopausal transition: evidence for accelerated loss and ultimate exhaustion. J Clin Endocrinol Metab. 1987;65(6):1231–7. https://doi.org/10.1210/jcem-65-6-1231. PMID: 3119654.

33. Wallace WH, Thomson AB, Kelsey TW. The radiosensitivity of the human oocyte. Hum Reprod. 2003;18(1):117–21. https://doi.org/10.1093/humrep/deg016. PMID: 12525451.

34. Wallace WH, Anderson R, Baird D. Preservation of fertility in young women treated for cancer. Lancet Oncol. 2004;5(5):269–70. https://doi.org/10.1016/S1470-2045(04)01462-7. PMID: 15120661.

35. Chang K, Merideth MA, Stratton P. Hormone use for therapeutic amenorrhea and contraception during hematopoietic cell transplantation. Obstet Gynecol. 2015;126(4):779–84. https://doi.org/10.1097/AOG.0000000000001031. PMID: 26348182; PMCID: PMC4580508.

36. Kirkham YA, Ornstein MP, Aggarwal A, McQuillan S. No. 313-menstrual suppression in special circumstances. J Obstet Gynaecol Can. 2019;41(2):e7–e17. https://doi.org/10.1016/j.jogc.2018.11.030. PMID: 30638562.

37. American College of Obstetricians and Gynecologists' Committee on Adolescent Health Care. Options for prevention and management of menstrual bleeding in adolescent patients undergoing cancer treatment: ACOG Committee Opinion, Number 817. Obstet Gynecol. 2021;137(1):e7–e15. https://doi.org/10.1097/AOG.0000000000004209. PMID: 33399429.

38. Poorvu PD, Barton SE, Duncan CN, London WB, Laufer MR, Lehmann LE, Marcus KJ. Use and effectiveness of gonadotropin-releasing hormone agonists for prophylactic menstrual sup-

pression in postmenarchal women who undergo hematopoietic cell transplantation. J Pediatr Adolesc Gynecol. 2016;29(3):265–8. https://doi.org/10.1016/j.jpag.2015.10.013. Epub 2015 Oct 23. PMID: 26506031.

39. Lhommé C, Brault P, Bourhis JH, Pautier P, Dohollou N, Dietrich PY, Akbar-Zadeh G, Lucas C, Pico JL, Hayat M. Prevention of menstruation with leuprorelin (GnRH agonist) in women undergoing myelosuppressive chemotherapy or radiochemotherapy for hematological malignancies: a pilot study. Leuk Lymphoma. 2001;42(5):1033–41. https://doi.org/10.3109/10428190109097723. PMID: 11697620.

40. Screening and management of bleeding disorders in adolescents with heavy menstrual bleeding: ACOG COMMITTEE OPINION, Number 785. Obstet Gynecol. 2019;134(3):e71–83. https://doi.org/10.1097/AOG.0000000000003411. PMID: 31441825.

41. ACOG committee opinion no. 557: management of acute abnormal uterine bleeding in nonpregnant reproductive-aged women. Obstet Gynecol. 2013;121(4):891–6. https://doi.org/10.1097/01.AOG.0000428646.67925.9a. PMID: 23635706.

42. Tsampras N, Gould D, Fitzgerald CT. Double ovarian stimulation (DuoStim) protocol for fertility preservation in female oncology patients. Hum Fertil. 2017;20(4):248–53.

43. Oktay K, Turan V, Bedoschi G, et al. Fertility preservation success subsequent to concurrent aromatase inhibitor treatment and ovarian stimulation in women with breast cancer. J Clin Oncol. 2015;33(22):2424–9.

44. Practice Committee of the American Society for Reproductive Medicine. Electronic address: asrm@asrm.org. Fertility preservation in patients undergoing gonadotoxic therapy or gonadectomy: a committee opinion. Fertil Steril. 2019;112(6):1022–33. https://doi.org/10.1016/j.fertnstert.2019.09.013. PMID: 31843073.

45. Diaz-Garcia C, Domingo J, Garcia-Velasco JA, Herraiz S, Mirabet V, Iniesta I, Cobo A, Remohí J, Pellicer A. Oocyte vitrification versus ovarian cortex transplantation in fertility preservation for adult women undergoing gonadotoxic treatments: a prospective cohort study. Fertil Steril. 2018;109(3):478–485.e2. https://doi.org/10.1016/j.fertnstert.2017.11.018. Epub 2018 Feb 7. PMID: 29428307.

46. Beckmann MW, Dittrich R, Lotz L, van der Ven K, van der Ven HH, Liebenthron J, Korell M, Frambach T, Sütterlin M, Schwab R, Seitz S, Müller A, von Wolff M, Häberlin F, Henes M, Winkler-Crepaz K, Krüssel JS, Germeyer A, Toth B. Fertility protection: complications of surgery and results of removal and transplantation of ovarian tissue. Reprod Biomed Online. 2018;36(2):188–96. https://doi.org/10.1016/j.rbmo.2017.10.109. Epub 2017 Nov 9. PMID: 29198423.

47. Irtan S, Orbach D, Helfre S, Sarnacki S. Ovarian transposition in prepubescent and adolescent girls with cancer. Lancet Oncol. 2013;14(13):e601–8. https://doi.org/10.1016/S1470-2045(13)70288-2. PMID: 24275133.

48. Gubbala K, Laios A, Gallos I, Pathiraja P, Haldar K, Ind T. Outcomes of ovarian transposition in gynaecological cancers; a systematic review and meta-analysis. J Ovarian Res. 2014;7:69. https://doi.org/10.1186/1757-2215-7-69. PMID: 24995040; PMCID: PMC4080752.

49. Caretto M, Simoncini T. The need to reduce gonadotoxicity! Fertility reserve after chemotherapy for gynaecological cancer. Gynecol Endocrinol. 2021;37(6):481–2. https://doi.org/10.1080/09513590.2021.1929153. Epub 2021 May 19.

50. Lambertini M, Horicks F, Del Mastro L, Partridge AH, Demeestere I. Ovarian protection with gonadotropin-releasing hormone agonists during chemotherapy in cancer patients: from biological evidence to clinical application. Cancer Treat Rev. 2019;72:65–77. https://doi.org/10.1016/j.ctrv.2018.11.006. Epub 2018 Dec 1. PMID: 30530271.

51. Oktay K, Harvey BE, Partridge AH, Quinn GP, Reinecke J, Taylor HS, Wallace WH, Wang ET, Loren AW. Fertility preservation in patients with cancer: ASCO clinical practice guideline update. J Clin Oncol. 2018;36(19):1994–2001. https://doi.org/10.1200/JCO.2018.78.1914. Epub 2018 Apr 5. PMID: 29620997.

52. Hyman JH, Tulandi T. Fertility preservation options after gonadotoxic chemotherapy. Clin Med Insights Reprod Health. 2013;7:61–9. https://doi.org/10.4137/CMRH.S10848. PMID: 24453520; PMCID: PMC3888081.

53. ESHRE Guideline Group on Female Fertility Preservation, Anderson RA, Amant F, Braat D, D'Angelo A, Chuva de Sousa Lopes SM, Demeestere I, Dwek S, Frith L, Lambertini M, Maslin C, Moura-Ramos M, Nogueira D, Rodriguez-Wallberg K, Vermeulen N. ESHRE guideline: female fertility preservation. Hum Reprod Open. 2020;2020(4):hoaa052. https://doi.org/10.1093/hropen/hoaa052. PMID: 33225079; PMCID: PMC7666361.

54. Lee JH, Choi YS. The role of gonadotropin-releasing hormone agonists in female fertility preservation. Clin Exp Reprod Med. 2021;48(1):11–26. https://doi.org/10.5653/cerm.2020.04049. Epub 2021 Feb 18. PMID: 33648041; PMCID: PMC7943347.

55. Floyd JL, Campbell S, Rauh-Hain JA, Woodard T. Fertility preservation in women with early-stage gynecologic cancer: optimizing oncologic and reproductive outcomes. Int J Gynecol Cancer. 2021;31(3):345–51. https://doi.org/10.1136/ijgc-2020-001328. Epub 2020 Jun 21. PMID: 32565487.

Premature Ovarian Insufficiency

Svetlana Vujovic, Miomira Ivovic, Milina Tancic Gajic, Ljiljana Marina, and Svetlana Dragojevic-Dikic

11.1 Introduction

Human life span has been significantly prolonged requiring early diagnosis and treating aging-related diseases. It is predicted that the number of people over 60 years old by 2050 will be five times that of 1950 [1]. One billion women will be menopausal in the next 25 years, and 80% of them will have some typical menopausal symptoms.

Quality of life is defined as the psychological and physical well-being depending on the influences of genetic and environmental factors.

Reproduction represents a biological key point necessary for the existence of the humankind during 20 million years on this planet. Adaptive mechanisms of women's bodies, influenced by many stressors, maintain homeostasis and reproductive potential. Chromosomes determine sex. Sex is biology. Nongonadal effects of sex chromosomes, coupled with gonadal effects through genomic actions, result in sex differentiation and gene expression in every cell. Nongonadal functions, directed by sex chromosomes, are critical for the physiology of organs (coagulation, energy metabolism, immunity, blood pressure, apoptosis, etc.). Gonadal steroids, estradiol, progesterone, testosterone, and others represent very important factors for maintaining homeostasis equilibrium. Low levels of gonadal and other steroid hormones have to be treated in order to avoid diseases.

S. Vujovic (✉) · M. Ivovic · M. Tancic Gajic · L. Marina
Faculty of Medicine, Clinic of Endocrinology, Diabetes and Diseases of Metabolism, University of Belgrade, University Clinical Center of Serbia, Belgrade, Serbia

S. Dragojevic-Dikic
Faculty of Medicine, Gynecology-Obstetrics Clinic Narodni Front, University of Belgrade, Belgrade, Serbia

© International Society of Gynecological Endocrinology 2023
A. R. Genazzani et al. (eds.), *Amenorrhea*, ISGE Series,
https://doi.org/10.1007/978-3-031-22378-5_11

11.2 Definition of POI

Fuller Albright, a Harvard endocrinologist, first described the condition called primary ovarian insufficiency [2]. Premature ovarian insufficiency (POI) is characterized by hypergonadotropic hypogonadism, oligo/amenorrhea with high gonadotropin, and low estradiol levels in women before 40 years of age. The most widely utilized diagnostic criterion for follicle-stimulating hormone (FSH) is >40 IU/mL [3]. Nelson RM et al. suggested FSH >30 IU/L [4] and the European Society of Human Reproduction and Embryology FSH >25 IU/L [5] on two occasions >4 weeks apart. Primary ovarian insufficiency describes a spectrum of declining ovarian functions and reduced fecundity due to a premature decrease in initial follicle number, an increase in follicle destruction, or poor follicular response to gonadotropins. It is not "the loss or cessation" of the ovarian activity since some significantly decreased level of ovarian activity is present in the whole life and extremely low number of follicles always remain. Possible induction of remaining follicle growth depends on the complete endocrine milieu. In order to achieve the more precise definition of decreasing levels of ovarian function, we suggest four grades of POI: grade I: FSH 10–20 IU/L; grade II: FSH 21–30 IU/L; grade III: FSH 31–40 IU/L; and grade IV: FSH >41 IU/L [6]. We suggest the earliest detection of ovarian insufficiency in order to initiate therapy on time.

11.3 Prevalence of POI

In the longitudinal cohort study involving 1858 women, Coulam CB et al. reported 1% prevalence of POI [7]. Luborsky JL et al. found differences between ethnic groups being the highest in US African-American and Hispanic women than Caucasian and lowest in Asian-American women [8]. A meta-analysis of the global prevalence of POI found a rate of 3.7% [9]. The prevalence of familial POI has been reported to be 4–31% in various studies [10, 11].

11.4 Etiology of POI

The etiology of POI still remains an enigma for many cases. Reduction in the primordial oocyte pool by accelerated follicular atresia, or destruction or problems in support, recruitment of maturated primordial or growing follicles can be the etiological factor.

The most prominent etiological factors causing POI can be divided into the following:

(A) **Primary**: Chromosome abnormalities, fragile X syndrome, gene polymorphism, autoimmune diseases, inhibin B mutations, enzyme deficiencies, and FSH receptor polymorphism.

Turner syndrome is an X-linked chromosomal abnormality involving the complete or partial loss of one X chromosome (deletions, translocations, inversions, isochromosomes, mosaicism). These women are usually born with a normal number of primordial follicles that undergo accelerated atresia [12].

Fragile X syndrome is characterized by premutation in the fragile X gene, mental retardation, and autism. 200 repeats of the CGG trinuclear repeat in gene 1 in the 5′ area of chromosome X are present.

Differences in gene-regulating pathways were found in Han Chinese vs. Serbian women in 8q22.3, HK3, and BRSK1 [13]. More genetic mutations have recently been discovered by whole-genome sequencing. In Table 11.1, some gene polymorphisms are shown. Differences between POI subgroups depending on the etiology were found.

None of the candidate genes is accepted as a genetic marker for POI.

POI may be induced by autoimmune antibodies and becomes a part of the inherited autoimmune condition caused by mutations in the autoimmune regulatory gene AIRE on chromosome 21.

Polyglandular autoimmune syndrome (PAI) comprises a diverse group of clinical conditions characterized by the functional impairment of multiple endocrine glands due to a loss of immune tolerance, described by Schmidt *1926* (Table 11.2). Abnormalities in self-recognition are present in 15% cases of premature ovarian insufficiency [14].

Table 11.1 Gene polymorphism in POI

Type	Gene	Locus
POI 1	FMR 1	Xq26-q28
POI 2A	DIAPH 2	Xq13.3-q21.1
POI 2B	POI 1B	Xq13.3-q21.1
POI 3	FOXL 2	3q23
POI 4	BMP 15	Xp11.2
POI 5	NOBOX	7q35
POI 6	FIGLA	2p12
POI 7	NR5 A1	9q33

Table 11.2 Autoimmune polyglandular syndrome and POI

Type	Inheritance	Autoimmune involvement	Age
I	Autosome recessive mutation in AIRE	Candidiasis Addison's disease Hypoparathyroidism	3–5 years
II	Polygenic dominant HLADR3	Addison's disease + Autoimmune thyroid disease (Schmidt) and/or diabetes mellitus type 1 (Carpenter syndrome)	III–IV decades
III	Apart from absence of adrenal failure	Hypothyroidism + other immune diseases with exclusion of Addison's disease	Adults

A part of autoimmune syndrome III is other autoimmune diseases like vitiligo, alopecia areata, diabetes mellitus type I, systemic lupus erythematosus, rheumatoid arthritis, and Sjogren's disease. Hypoestrogenism in POI directly decreases adaptive autoimmune response and can induce autoimmune diseases. Activated T lymphocytes are decreased, autoimmunity is enhanced, effector helper T lymphocytes and macrophages are activated, and production of potentially protective B cells is diminished [15]. While Kirshenbaum M et al. found the most significant association of POI with adrenal insufficiency (2.5–20%) [16], we found autoimmune lymphocyte Hashimoto's thyroiditis in 27% of POI and only 2% of Addison's diseases in a group of 2000 POI women. Our findings were in concordance with the finding of Bunpei I that POI was associated with hypothyroidism most frequently, followed by hyperparathyroidism [17].

Hypoestrogenism increases obesity promoting autoimmune diseases by the following mechanisms:

1. Vitamin D deficiency, increased B cells, antibody production, T helper 17 decrease
2. Microbiome alteration increases T helper 17 and decreases T regulatory lymphocytes
3. Increase of inhibitory macrophage apoptosis, NLRP3, interleukin-1-beta, and interleukin-18; inflammasome activation
4. Decrease of natural killer cells and T regulatory lymphocytes, leading to inflammation, and increase of T helper 17 lymphocytes

Metabolic causes include the following:

I. Deficiency of 17 hydroxylase: increased levels of FSH, luteinizing hormone (LH), deoxycorticosterone, progesterone, hypertension, alkalosis with high potassium

II. Deficiency of galactose-1 phosphate uridyltransferase: intracellular accumulation of galactose metabolites and deficiency of granulosa cell pool

(B) **Secondary**: bilateral oophorectomy, chemotherapy, uterine artery embolization, infections

Iatrogenic cases occurred following ovarian surgery in 64 and 88% due to cystectomy. Mean period of the onset of ovarian insufficiency after ovarian surgery was 5.8 + 3.8 years [18]. The commonest chemotherapies, including cyclophosphamide, cisplatin, doxorubicin, anthracyclines, alkylating agents, and allogenic stem cell transplants, cause more than 90% POI [19]. Polycyclic aromatic hydrocarbon exposure, cigarette smoking, exposure to phthalates, bisphenol A, and other environmental pollutants can be associated with POI.

The most frequent infections inducing POI are mumps, varicella, and tuberculosis.

11.5 Pathogenesis of POI

Spontaneous POI can be a part of an early aging syndrome in some women. Epigenetic aging can begin a few weeks postconception in fetal tissues [20].

In 2009, the Nobel Prize in Physiology or Medicine was awarded to Dr. Blackburn EH, Szostak JW, and Greider CW for the explanation on how chromosomes are protected by telomere and the enzyme telomerase. Telomerases are responsible for the synthesis of chromosomal DNA ends. A significant association was found between shortening of telomerase repeats upon successive cell division, limiting viability, and ending with cell death and a reduction of the replicative life span of cultured human cells, consistent with the early genetic evidence that short telomeres induce senescence. Introduction of telomerase into the normal human cells extends life span [21]. Mutations in genes encoding components of the telomerase complex cause hereditary disease characterized by defects in the stem cell renewal and tissue maintenance. Stressors triggering POI can influence telomerase and accelerate biological clock. In our study, performed on 2000 POI patients, stressor was a triggering factor in 56% of cases. Divorce or separation from the partner was the most prominent stressor. Stress, as a disease, develops when adaptive mechanisms are broken under the influences of too strong stressors or stressors of too long duration [22].

In such a disbalance of homeostasis and loss of adaptive mechanism, resistance, and resilience, POI is in correlation with the inflammatory aging. Oxidative stress refers to an imbalance between oxidation and antioxidation leading to neutrophil infiltrations. Increase in interleukin-6, interleukin-8, interleukin-1β, interleukin-10, tissue growth factor beta (TGFß), interferon γ, and prostaglandin E_2 and decrease of tumor necrosis factor α and interleukin-2 were detected in POI. Antioxidants help organisms to fight against free radicals. They can be divided into two groups:

– *Enzymatic*: superoxide dismutase, catalase, glutathione peroxidase, transferase, thiol-disulfide oxidoreductase
– *Nonenzymatic*: transferrin, ferritin, lactoferrin, hemoglobin, albumin, glutathione, ascorbic acid, A-tocopherol, ubiquinone, beta-carotene, uric acid, bilirubin

Decreased gamma-glutamyl transpeptidase and diacron reactive oxygen metabolite were found, while C-reactive protein was increased. DNA damage continues to accumulate leading to cell death in POI. Autophagic cleansing capacity declines gradually. Dysfunctional protein accumulation in mitochondria increases the level of reactive oxygen species and oxidative stress [23]. Resveratrol restores ovarian function by increasing AMH and decreasing inflammation through upregulation of expression of the peroxisome proliferator-activator receptor and SIRT1 (sirtuin 1) inhibiting interferon γ-induced inflammatory cytokines [24].

11.6   Clinical Symptoms and Signs

11.6.1   Early Symptoms and Signs

Typical symptoms and signs of POI are hot flushes, night sweats, irritability, anxiety, depression, mood swings, loss of concentration, insomnia, loss of libido, vaginal dryness, dyspareunia, gaining of weight, etc.

11.6.2   Late Symptoms and Signs

Late symptoms and signs of untreated POI include cardiovascular diseases (impaired endothelial dysfunction, ischemic heart disease, myocardial infarction, etc.), metabolic syndrome, diabetes mellitus, osteoporosis, bone fractures, cognitive impairments, urogenital and sexual disorders, infertility, lower quality of life, and twofold age-specific mortality rate [25].

11.7   Complications of Untreated POI

11.7.1   Cardiovascular Diseases

William Harvey's discovery that heart pumps blood and the blood circulates (1628) was fundamental for later understanding that gonadal steroids are bound to the receptors in blood vessels. Also, estradiol receptors are found in cardiomyocytes, fibroblasts, and endothelial cells, and progesterone receptors in cardiomyocytes, vascular smooth muscle cells, and endothelial cells.

In a group of 144,260 amenorrheic women, included in the study of Honigberg MC, 4904 (3.4%) had spontaneous POI and 644 (0.4%) had surgical POI. The primary outcome occurred in 292 (6.0%) women with spontaneous POI (8.78/1000 woman-years) and 49 (7.6%) women with surgical POI (11.27/1000 woman-years) compared to 5415 (3.9%) menopausal women (5.70/1000 woman-years). For the primary outcome, spontaneous and surgical POI was associated with HRs of 1.36 (95% CI 1.19–1.56; $p < 0.001$) and 1.87 (95% CI 1.36–2.58; $p < 0.001$), respectively, after adjusting for cardiovascular disease risk factors and menopausal hormone therapy usage [26]. In Table 11.3, mortality rate in untreated POI is presented [27–34].

Hypoestrogenism exerts effects on many levels: lipids, insulin resistance, obesity, inflammation, hypertension, vasoconstriction, endothelial dysfunction, autonomic nervous system dysfunction, nitric oxide disturbances, impaired flow-mediated dilatation [35], etc. Benefits of early initiation of estroprogestogens have been confirmed in many recent trials and meta-analyses. The dose and type of hormones at the initiation of therapy appeared crucial for obtaining coronary heart disease benefits [36].

Patients with POI have to be provided with adequate information about the therapy. They should maintain a healthy lifestyle, balanced diet, physical activity, and good sleeping habits and avoid smoking.

Table 11.3 Mortality rate in untreated POI

Name	Observation	Number	Years
Van der Schouw YT [27]	Cardiovascular mortality was decreased 2% for every year menopause is delayed	12,000	20
Tao XY [28]	48% higher risk for ischemic heart diseases in POI		
Rahman H [29]	Earlier menopause (40–45 years of age) increase 40% risk for ischemic heart disease, compared with menopause at 50s		
Van Lennep JER [30]	10 observational studies, with 9440 events, showed that POI is an independent risk factor for IHD	190,588	
Amaghai Y [31]	Higher mortality rate in POI in Japan	3824	9
Gallagher LG [32]	Higher mortality rate in POI in China	267,400	
Jacobsen BK [33]	Higher mortality rate in POI in Norway	1973	20
Wu X et al. [34]	Higher mortality rate in POI	1003	

11.7.2 Metabolic Changes

Estradiol regulates many of the key enzymes involved in mitochondrial bioenergetics including glucose transporters, required for the regulation of glucose uptake in cells and tissues. GLUT4 is regulated by insulin receptor Akt/TOR signaling network. Disturbances in insulin metabolism in the endometrium decrease endometrium receptivity and fertility rate and trigger obesity, insulin resistance, and diabetes mellitus later in the life. Adipocyte hypertrophy, adipose tissue inflammation, fat liver, and changes of glucose uptake from the circulation, without changes in "de novo" free fatty acid synthesis, create redistribution of body fat to centripetal, metabolic type. Kulaksizoglu M et al. found increased serum glucose and insulin through homeostasis model assessment for insulin resistance (HOMA) in POI patients with hypoestrogenism [37].

Tissue resistance to insulin increases the risk of developing coronary heart disease and type 2 diabetes mellitus. Hypoestrogenism leads to weight increase of 5 kg and redistribution of fatty tissue to a more central type, leading to metabolic syndrome.

Decreased dehydroepiandrosterone (DHEA) and dehydroepiandrosterone sulfate (DHEAS) in POI patients result in increased ratio of cortisol to DHEA creating "cortisol-potentiated diseases": obesity, insulin resistance, diabetes mellitus type 2, osteoporosis, neurodegeneration, etc.

11.7.3 Osteoporosis

Estradiol deficiency increase bone loss increasing osteoclast formation (activated T lymphocyte cells), differentiation and recruitment to the bone surface, prolonging osteoclast life span and increases erosion depth, proinflammatory cytokines production IL-7 and tissue necrosis factor alfa (TNFα). Hypoestrogenism in POI induces excessive production of the cytokine receptor activator of nuclear factor kappa β ligand (RANKL) by osteoblasts, which stimulates osteoclastogenesis and bone resorption leading to osteoporosis. The incidence of hip fracture in POI was 9.4% compared to 3.3% in those entering menopause at the age of 48 years [38]. Meczekalski B et al. found that hypoestrogenism and hypoandrogenism have deleterious effects on peak bone mass formation and bone mineral density [39].

FSH is in positive correlation with skeletal bone density. Lana et al. reported that serum FSH concentrations, but not estradiol concentrations, are positively associated with bone mass loss in skeletal regions (both the spinal column and femoral neck) in patients with spontaneous POI [40]. In Popat VB et al.'s study of 32-year-old POI patients, significantly decreased BMD was found. In 21% of patients, Z-score was −2.8 and in 67% femoral Z-score was <−1.0 [41]. Recently performed study on 200 idiopathic POI and 200 POI with bilateral oophorectomy showed that Z-score is significantly lower in POI patients, compared to controls (Z-score −2.26). Patients with bilateral adnexectomy had significantly lower Z-score. Estradiol <32 pg/mL was in correlation with loss of bone mineral density. Idiopathic POI showed preserved BMD for 3 years, osteopenia was found from 5 to 7 amenorrheic years, and osteoporosis was observed after that [42].

11.7.4 Cognitive Health and Brain Function

Two-third of brain weight is blood vessels with receptors for estradiol, progesterone, and androgens. Estradiol is involved in all brain functions and studies done at the level of hippocampus, striatum, and prefrontal cortex controlling language abilities, verbal fluences, memory, sleeping, learning, and evaluation process. Estradiol influences neuroprotection at the levels of cerebral microvascularization, mitochondria, anti-inflammation, synaptic plasticity, neurogenesis, cholinergic neurotransmission, cellular maintenance, and survival. Declining short-term memory and cognitive function and increased incidence of Alzheimer's disease have been reported in patients with POI, but these phenomena have not been observed before or after the age-appropriate menopause. Oophorectomy before the age of menopause increases the risk of cognitive impairment or dementia nearly twofold [43].

Rocca WA et al., using data from the Mayo Clinic, studied oophorectomy and aging on 813 women with unilateral adnexectomy, 676 with bilateral oophorectomy, and 1472 controls. They found that women who underwent surgery before the age of natural menopause had an increase of cognitive impairment or dementia compared to controls [44].

These data suggest that early estrogen deficiency has deleterious effects on the brain and correlates with nervousness, anxiety, depression, irritability, lack of concentration, insomnia, restlessness, etc. in POI.

11.7.5   Urogenital Function and Sexuality

Vaginal dryness, painful intercourse, vulvar pruritus, burning and discomfort, and recurrent urogenital infections are induced by hypoestrogenic effects on vagina, vulva, bladder, and urethral epithelium and changes in pH [45].

POI patients showed worse sex performance with more pain and poorer lubrication than controls, suggesting that estrogen and testosterone therapy can be useful in reestablishing epithelium cells, vaginal pH, and microflora.

Changes in body shape, body image concerns, gaining of weight, and psychological changes may impair the sense of attractiveness. Young age and distressing impact of such a life-changing as well as symptomatic vulvovaginal atrophy and hypoactive sexual desire modulate central and peripheral sexual response [46]. Hypoestrogenism influences sexual pathways and increases the risk of sexual dysfunction two- to eightfold in POI [47].

11.7.6   Infertility

Information that oocyte donation is the only option for fertility in women with POI makes them shocked, devastated, feel worthless, and confused. Is it really the truth? It is not always the only truth, and we have to be more empathetic to POI patients. They should be informed that there is a small chance for spontaneous pregnancy, or medically supported pregnancy. As well, they have to be reassured that their pregnancy will not show any higher obstetric or pathological risk than in general population.

In the menopausal women 1 year after the last menstruation, about 1000 oocytes are still present in the ovaries. Some of them are of good quality but most are not. Successful pregnancy rate after in vitro fertilization (IVF) with oocyte donation is not optimal due to underdiagnosed endometrial endocrine, immunological, and hematological disorders.

Van Kesteren YM et al. showed that nearly three out of four women with POI have ovarian follicles remaining in the ovary [48]. Study of Letru-Konirsch H et al. showed that endometrium previously prepared with adequate doses of estradiol and progesterone combined with pentoxifylline and tocopherol resulted in 30–50% pregnancies with fresh embryos and 15–25% with frozen thawed embryos [49]. Conventional substitution of estradiol in POI is not sufficient for inducing dominant follicle growth and adequate endometrial responsiveness. In order to create optimal endocrine milieu for remaining follicle growth, we suggest higher doses of estradiol trying to decrease FSH to 10–15 IU/L [50]. Clinical study on 376 POI patients with pregnancy rates of 18% allowed us to suggest the following: In a case that during 6 months no dominant follicles were obtained and FSH value was 10–15 IU/L (day 2), the best solution was oocyte donation. Well-estrogenized brain of POI women allowed them to accept this solution even more having in mind that all other tissues are well prepared, especially endometrium.

Estradiol actions are mediated via genomic and nongenomic pathways. Estradiol receptor alpha promotes mitogenic activation and proliferation, while ERβ protects endometrium from the undesired action of ERα. It improves vascularization and endometrial flow; sensitizes and differentiates granulosa cells; stimulates endometrial proliferation, myometrium receptivity, and production of the cervical mucus; and directly influences immune response. Estradiol receptors are expressed in various lymphoid tissue cells, lymphocytes, macrophages, and dendritic cells.

Estradiol downregulates FSH receptors and luteinizing hormone receptors. It increases the response of FSH and number of LH receptors previously induced by FSH. One of the important estradiol therapy goals is to decrease the high endogenous FSH. Chronic elevation of FSH downregulates granulosa FSH receptors. Premature ovarian insufficiency is not a failure but rather an intermittent and unpredictable ovarian function that can persist for decades. Tonic elevation of LH causes premature luteinization of growing antral follicles [51]. Estroprogestogen therapy may restore FSH receptors and may enhance the ability of ovarian follicles to avoid premature luteinization.

Optimal concentrations of estradiol and progesterone are crucial for early steps of embryo implantation and development. Successful implantation requires mother-embryo cross talk and coordination of embryo development with endometrium receptors. Four major phases of endometrium transformation make transcriptome signature. Preimplantation inhibitory factors were secreted in 77.6% of all successful implantation. Estradiol/progesterone ratio plays a critical role in embryo receptivity by the endometrium. Hyperinsulinism decreases the number of insulin receptors, IGF-1 receptors, IGFBP-1 receptors, and SHBG. PAI-1 inhibits plasminogen activators and fibrinolysis and potentiates thromboembolic effect. Stressors induce the increase of corticotropin-releasing hormone (CRH), adrenocorticotropin hormone (ACTH), prolactin, and cortisol and decrease prostaglandin, E2 release, angiotensin II, nitric oxide, acetylcholine, and serotonin-potentiated vasoconstriction. Also, growth hormone and thyroid hormone are required [52].

Trypsin, a serin protease, released by preimplantation embryos, elicits Ca 2^+ signaling in endometrial epithelial cells. Competent human embryos trigger short-lived oscillatory Ca 2^+ fluxes inducing genes involved in implantation and postimplantation development. Low-quality embryos caused a heightened and prolonged Ca 2^+ response. The decidualizing endometrium secretes serine protease inhibitors to limit embryo-derived proteolytic activity. The acquisition of the secretory phenotype upon decidualization depends on the massive expansion of estrogen receptors [53].

Insulin resistance and hyperinsulinism induce obesity and increase androgens and plasminogen activator inhibitor. It decreases glycodelin, insulin-like growth factor-binding protein 1 (IGFBP 1), and uterus vascularity, decreasing endometrium receptivity.

As well, thyroid function has to be tested. Suggested TSH value is 1–2.5 mmol/L in order to prepare endometrium for embryo implantation. During any kind of therapy for thyroid gland (hyper- or hypothyroidism), TSH has to be detected once monthly. Also, detection of antinuclear antibodies, anticardiolipin antibodies, and thrombophilia (Leiden V, FII, MTHFR, PAI mutations) is suggested in order to improve endometrium receptivity and prevent miscarriages.

DHEA is converted to estradiol, which suppresses FSH. Increase of testosterone production by early follicles stimulates androgen receptors allowing more preantral follicles to progress to more mature antral follicles [54]. It induces antral follicle growth and increases follicle sensitivity to gonadotropins and endometrium receptivity. A Cochrane systemic review concluded that DHEA and its derivate testosterone may improve live birth rates.

Ovarian tissue cryopreservation can be performed in prepubertal girls at risk of POI. This procedure is feasible and safe compared to other operative procedures in children [55].

Receptors for melatonin are present on theca cells. Three times higher melatonin concentration was found in preovulatory follicle compared to serum concentration. In the presence of human chorionic gonadotropin, melatonin has a putative role decreasing cAMP, estradiol, and progesterone in preovulatory follicle. It inhibits gonadotropin-releasing hormone (GnRH), decreases response of LH to LHRH, increases GABA and prolactin, prolongs cortisol peak during the night, and inhibits TSH and growth hormone. The study of Dragojevic Dikic S. showed favorable effects of melatonin on the fertility rate in POI women [56].

11.8 Diagnosis of POI

- **History taking** (menarche, menstrual regularities, oligo/amenorrhea, hot flushes, mood swings, anxiety, depression, loss of concentration, insomnia, loss of libido, dyspareunia, etc.).
- **Analysis**: Blood count, glycemia, lipid profile, liver analysis, electrolyte status, HgbA1c.
- **Hormones**: FSH, LH, estradiol, AMH, inhibin B, prolactin, free thyroxin, thyroid-stimulating hormone (TSH), free testosterone, androstenedione, DHEAS, vitamin D.
- **Thrombophilia and immunological testing**: Leyden V, FII, MTHFR, PAI, antinuclear antibodies, anticardiolipin antibodies, anti-TPO, anti-TG, lupus anticoagulants.
- **Oral glucose tolerance test** (OGTT) is performed after 12-h starvation at 8 am with 75 g of glucose orally ingested, and measurement of glucose and insulin on 30-min interval during 2 h has to be done. HOMA index is less sensitive and specific compared with area under the curve, calculated in OGTT for testing insulin sensitivity.
- **Ultrasound** of thyroid gland, breasts, abdomen, uterus, and ovaries (total ovary volume, antral follicle count).
- **Karyotype**, especially for younger than 30 years of age.
- **Osteodensitometry (DEXa)** for those who are not planning pregnancy soon.

AMH can be undetectable 5 years before periods cease. No diagnostic cutoffs have been established, but it is used as one of the diagnostic tools for POI [57]. It appears to be a stronger predictor of ovarian response to gonadotropin therapy than antral follicle count in assisted reproduction treatment.

11.9   Differential Diagnosis

The most important differential diagnosis is resistant ovary syndrome, characterized by elevated FSH, LH, normal AMH, and antral follicle count. The ovaries are unresponsive to endogenous and exogenous FSH due to genetic or immunological inactivation of FSH or LH receptor [58].

11.10   Therapy of POI

Hormone therapy in POI patients facilitates the development of secondary sexual characteristics (including uterine growth in prepubertal girls with primary amenorrhea). Barriga PP et al. suggested in a case that no spontaneous menarche occurs and elevated FSH is detected in children 12–13 years of age therapy with 17ß-estradiol (E_2) has to be initiated transdermally 6.25 µg/day E_2 via patch or transdermal aerosol: 3.16 mg mg/day or gel 0.5–1.5 mg/day, or oral micronized E_2: 5 µg/kg/day, or E_2 valerate 0.25 mg/day. Gradual increase of therapy with 6-month intervals is suggested. After 2 years of estradiol therapy, or when breakthrough bleeding occurs, cyclical progestogen has to be initiated during 10–14 days of the month: oral medroxyprogesterone acetate 5–10 mg/day, or oral micronized progesterone 100–200 mg/day, or dydrogesterone 5–10 mg/day, or nomegestrol acetate 5–10 mg/day, or desogestrel [59].

Hormone replacement therapy alleviates typical symptoms, improves quality of life, creates favorable hormonal environment for pregnancy, and minimizes long-term effects. Replaced hormones should be identical to those that are missing. The aim of estroprogestogen therapy would be to achieve relatively physiological levels of estradiol (200–400 pmol/L). Non/oral estrogen delivery routes offer advantages in regard to avoiding first-pass hepatic metabolism and minimizing prothrombotic effects. The estrogen doses should be generally higher than used in natural menopause. Combined oral contraceptives may be used until the expected time of the menopause [60].

The role of progestogens in the therapy of POI is very often advised only to women with uterus. We would like to accentuate that progesterone receptors A and B are present in all blood vessels inducing many changes from the brain to all other tissues. Progestogens balance with estrogens and imitate "natural cycles." Confusion arose due to usage of different kinds of progestogens in therapy. Today, we prefer to use natural progestogens vaginally, orally, and transdermally. Micronized progesterone is superior for insulin resistance and HDL improvement. Vaginal micronized progesterone may have the benefit of achieving higher levels within the uterus with lower doses compared to oral.

Other therapy regimens in POI patients include testosterone, DHEAS, melatonin, metformin, myoinositol, L-carnitine, etc. The free radical theory of aging describes that oxidative stress leads to changes in the ovarian microenvironment and these changes account for the ovarian senescence and decrease of ovarian reserve.

Vitamin C, N-acetyl-L-cysteine, curcumin, coenzyme Q, proanthocyanidin, caloric restriction mimetics, regulators of glycolytic metabolism, inhibitors of insulin/ IGF-1 signaling pathway, inhibitors of mTOR pathway, epigenetic regulators (small molecule inhibit DNA methylation and histone acetyltransferases or noncoding RNAs), sirtuin activators and resveratrol, microRNAs, telomerase activators were suggested in some studies [61].

Nonhormonal pharmacological options (paroxetine, venlafaxine, gabapentin, oxybutynin, and clonidine) should be advised only for the alleviation of vasomotor symptoms where hormone therapy is contraindicated. Myoinositol, in combination with other therapeutic modalities, additionally improves fertility rate in POI [62].

11.10.1 Cardiovascular Effects

Estradiol therapy has antioxidative effects, by increasing the levels of endothelial nitric oxide synthase and production of nitric oxide regulating blood pressure, platelet function, vascular smooth muscle proliferation, and expression of adhesion molecules. It reduces the release of endothelin-1, a potent vasoconstrictor, exerting anti-inflammatory effects on blood vessels. Estradiol therapy improves arterial function, heart rate variability, and baroreceptor sensitivity. It modulates arrhythmia vulnerability. Slopes are more steeper, and QT dynamics are impaired in POI. Canpolat U et al. showed that therapy with 17β-estradiol could exert an antiarrhythmic effect by inhibition of Ca^{2+} channels [63]. Data obtained with ambulatory blood pressure monitoring on transdermal estradiol and drospirenone are concordant with definitively positive effects on blood pressure compared to control group.

Secondary hypertension in POI can be induced by:

1. Low estradiol levels, changed ratio of E2/testosterone
2. Genes (renin-angiotensin system, adrenergic system, eNOS, adducin-1, estrogen-related aromatase)
3. Relative hyperaldosteronism inducing prothrombotic activity, endothelial dysfunction, autonomous nervous system dysfunction

Daan NMP et al. [64] found decreased glomerular filtration rate in POI. Estradiol therapy increases natrium excretion, improves baroreceptor function, prevents vascular fibrosis, improves diastolic function, decreases blood pressure and ventricular ectopic activity, inhibits mitochondrial reactive oxygen species in cardiomyocytes, and decreases mortality rate from ischemic heart failure. Goldmeier S found significantly lower catalase and superoxide dismutase, markers of autonomous dysfunction in POI. It changes heart rate variability, baroreceptor sensitivity, and dispersion of repolarization [65]. The National Institute of Health's study of transdermal estrogens 100 µg/day with medroxyprogesterone acetate 10 mg/day during 12 days monthly showed decrease in cardiovascular risk factors, including LDL levels, fibrinogen, and blood pressure [66].

11.10.2 Metabolic Effects

Estrogen therapy has beneficial effects on the metabolism of glycose improving insulin sensitivity. Oral estrogen effects are more pronounced compared with transdermal estrogen. These effects can be impaired by addition of androgenic progestogens (norgestrel, medroxyprogesterone acetate), while nonandrogenic progestogens do not have these unwanted effects. Estroprogestogen therapy reverses changes of body fat distribution by increasing the levels of endothelial nitric oxide synthase and production of nitric oxide. It regulates eating behavior, increases lipolytic adrenalin effects, decreases oxygen peptides, and protects from hepatic steatosis.

Hyperinsulinism increases LH directly in the pituitary. Treating insulin resistance with metformin alters energy metabolism in cells. It lowers glucose levels by inhibiting hepatic gluconeogenesis and opposing the actions of glucagon. The primary site of metformin action is mitochondria. The inhibition of mitochondrial complex I of the electron transport chain induces drop in energy charge, resulting in adenosine triphosphate (ATP) decrease. Adenosine monophosphate (AMP) increases bounding of P-site adenylate cyclase enzyme leading to defective cAMP protein kinase A (CAMPK) signaling on glucagon receptor. AMPK is an energy sensor and a master coordinator of an integrated signaling network that comprises metabolic growth pathways acting in synchrony to restore cellular energy balance. They switch on catabolic pathways that generate ATP and switch off anabolic pathways. Stimulation of 5'-AMP-activated protein kinase confers insulin sensitivity, mainly by modulating lipid metabolism. Metformin increases glucose uptake in skeletal muscles. It blocks insulin receptor/R/3K/Akt/mTOR signaling in the hyperplastic endometrial tissue inducing GLUT4 expression and inhibiting androgen receptor expression [67].

Metformin suppresses food intake by increasing the levels of glucagon-like peptide 1 and interaction with ghrelin and leptin on the T cell memory by altering fatty acid metabolism [68].

Insulin resistance, with increasing LH in the menopause, participates in adrenal tumorigenesis showing us that early detection and treatment of insulin resistance can be protective for many diseases [69].

11.10.3 Osteoporosis

Ethinyl estradiol has a more potent effect on bone markers. It suppresses gonadotropins profoundly. Estradiol may be preferable to the combined oral contraceptive pill (COCP) in women with POI with regard to the bone health (increased bone formation and decreased resorption). Therapy with estradiol increases osteoprotegerin (OPG), secreted by osteoblasts, which inhibits RANKL [41].

Therapy with 100 μg/day of transdermal estradiol and 10 mg MPA during 10 days monthly during 3 years makes no differences compared to bone mineral density in normally cycling control group. Prompt treatment of POI with estroprogestogens prevents osteoporosis and fractures. Bisphosphonates are not indicated in

POI patients. Given the extremely long half-life of bisphosphonates, there is concern regarding the safety of this class of drugs in POI planning pregnancy [70]. Low bone mass in women with primary ovarian insufficiency is managed most appropriately with HT.

11.10.4 Brain Effects

Luine FN et al. found that estradiol promotes neuronal growth, survival, transmission, myelinization, neural plasticity, dendritic branching, function, and synaptogenesis and improves cognitive function [43]. Cognitive decline and increased incidence of Alzheimer's diseases in women with early age at surgical menopause were found in a study of Bove R et al. [71]. Estroprogestogen therapy reduces the possible risk of cognitive impairment.

11.10.5 Sexuality

Sexual problems cannot be completely resolved only by estroprogestogen therapy in majority of women [45]. Estrogen therapy maintains vaginal elasticity and optimal length. In reproductive years, endogenous production of testosterone is 300 μg daily (50% by ovaries and 50% by adrenal glands). It is advised in women with hypoactive sexual desire and bilateral adnexectomy. Testosterone has an initiating role in desire and central arousal, acting on the dopaminergic tone and modulating peripheral actions as a permitting factor for nitric oxide, the main mediator of clitoral and cavernosal bodies' congestion. Both estrogens and androgens influence brain and genitourinary physiology requiring both hormones in therapy for well sexual functioning [46]. With 30 years' experience with testosterone gels in Europe, transdermal testosterone for women can be added to those with hypoactive sexual desire and adnexectomy. It is very important for feelings of well-being, energy, and sexuality. Meta-analysis of testosterone levels performed in different types of spontaneous POI, including 529 women compared to 319 controls, showed that POI women had significantly lower testosterone levels than controls [72]. They require a physiological dose of 5 mg/day (compared to 50 mg/day in men).

Wong QHY et al. showed beneficial effects of DHEA supplementation during 12 months in POI [73].

There were insufficient data to make a recommendation for the use of oral DHEA to improve female sexual desire by recent global consensus position statement [74].

11.10.6 Infertility

Natural or modified cycles with estroprogestogens represent first-line therapy with the aim to decrease FSH from 10 to 15 IU/L [50]. Low-dose human chorionic gonadotropins can be advised in grade I POI [75].

Higher estradiol dose therapy, with progesterone in the luteal phase, restores normal ovulatory activity, increases oocyte and egg quality, increases fertilization rate, proposes selective serotonin reuptake receptor-like role and growth and survival of cells, and increases insulin sensitivity and HDL.

With increasing estradiol doses in order to induce follicle growth, our team confirmed higher rate of pregnancy than usually referred (5%) at 18% [76]. It is important to stress that contraception can be achieved with hormone menopause therapy but at the age of natural menopause, not 2 years after initiating therapy.

Clomiphene citrate has no proven benefits.

Depending on immunological and hematological findings, methylfolate, aspirin, and pronison can be added in therapy. During pregnancy, depending on D-dimer, low-molecular-weight heparin is advised.

Other therapeutic modalities include prednisone (4 × 25 mg 4 weeks) for autoimmune POI, plasmapheresis in myasthenia gravis, pentoxifylline-tocopherol, apoptotic inhibitors, sphingosine 1-phosphate, autotransplantation, and xenotransplantation.

Ljubic A et al. showed principles of autologous ovarian in vitro activation with ultrasound-guided orthotopic re-transplantation [77]. Rosatio R and Anderson RA described the activation of residual primordial follicles and therapy with platelet-rich plasma [78]. Folliculogenesis was detected in women with POI treated with mesenchymal stem cells extracted from bone merrow, peripheral blood mononuclear cells, adipose tissue, placenta, umbilical cord, and menstrual blood.

Meta-analysis of 24 papers, on 892 women with pelvic irradiation due to malignancies who had ovarian transposition, showed significant preservation rate. Adult ovaries preserve rare numbers of oogonial stem cells that can stably proliferate for months and produce mature oocytes in vitro. Injection of labeled OSCs into mouse ovaries leads to differentiation of these cells into mature oocytes that are ovulated and fertilized and generate viable neonates [79]. Liu et al. showed that mesenchymal stem cell properties and in vivo survival of human endometrial stem cells make them ideal seed cells for stem cell transplantation in the treatment of POI [80]. A Cochrane systemic review concluded that DHEA and its derivate testosterone may improve live birth rates.

11.11 Risks of HRT and POI

11.11.1 Breast Cancer

HRT does not affect breast density in women with spontaneous POI [81]. In a systemic review of 15 publications addressing this question, 5 demonstrated an association between oral contraceptive pill use of at least 5–10 years and breast cancer, whereas the remaining 10 demonstrated no such association [82]. Meta-analyses have demonstrated no association between long-term oral contraceptive pill use and breast cancer risk when pooling estimates of multiple studies [83]. Other studies confirm the absence of an increased risk for breast cancer in women with POI taking

HRT [84]. Only combined regimens should be used in women with POI and an intact uterus, although as this is so well established in women with natural menopause there are no studies specifically addressing this in women with POI. In young women with POI, Gordhandas S et al. showed the benefits of prophylactic risk-reducing bilateral salpingo-oophorectomy in women carrying the BRCA1 and -2 genes, which do not appear to be mitigated when HT is added back as long as the individual does not have a past history of hormone receptor-positive breast cancer [85]. Latest studies of Carroll J showed that progesterone receptors and androgen receptors impinge estrogen receptors' transcriptional activity, and cross talk between different nuclear receptors is important [86]. This observation markedly supports the importance of adding progesterone, and, when necessary, androgens to women after hysterectomy during the menopause. Hyperinsulinism in hypoestrogenic environment during the menopause additionally lowers progesterone levels and can trigger breast carcinoma in patients with genetic predispositions. Our attention has to be paid to decreasing insulin levels in POI and natural menopause.

11.11.2   Stroke, Venous Thromboembolism

The absolute risk for stroke is extremely low, with no studies on the effect of HRT treatment. Only one study assessed the risks of venous thromboembolism (VTE) in women with POI, finding no significant association between first VTE and HRT use. Estrogen therapy should be delivered transdermally in women thought to be at increased risk, as first pass is avoided, mainly in women with natural menopause [87]. Transdermal is the preferred route for delivery of estradiol in women with POI at increased risk of VTE. Those with prior VTE or a thrombophilic disorder can be referred to a hematologist prior to commencing HRT.

11.11.3   Endometriosis

Endometriosis is a lifelong, inborn, autoimmune disease. Estroprogestogen therapy in the POI is needed. As it is an estrogen-dependent disease, the use of estrogen replacement therapy in women with endometriosis and POI (for instance, after hysterectomy and adnexectomy) could theoretically reactivate residual disease, produce new lesions, or even lead to malignant transformation of endometriosis. Dunselman et al. suggested oophorectomy as an option for improving pain related to endometriosis [88]. However, endometriotic tissue can be found anywhere in the body. Our suggestion is estroprogestogen therapy in all women with POI. In our group of women with endometriosis and POI, no increasing endometriotic cysts or neoplasm was found in a group of 648 women. Continuous combined estrogen/progestogen therapy can be effective for the treatment of vasomotor symptoms and may reduce the risk of endometriosis reactivation after oophorectomy.

11.11.4 Migraine

Migraine is not a contraindication for HRT use in women with POI. Changing dose, route of administration, or regimen may help if migraine worsens during HRT. Transdermal delivery may be the lowest-risk route of administration of estrogen for migraine sufferers with aura.

11.11.5 Fibroids

Two systematic reviews of postmenopausal women showed no significant increase in clinical symptoms or adverse effects associated with fibroid growth after HRT use [89]. Fibroids are not a contraindication to HRT use by women with POI.

11.12 Conclusion

Individual approach is necessary, and yearly hormone level control is necessary in order to optimize dosages in POI patients. Hormone therapy is not age limited and can be lifelong. It has to be individually tailored, with appropriate dosages and route of administration [90]. Excluding estroprogestogen therapy after the age of 55 abruptly increases cardiovascular diseases in the first year of discontinuation. After the age of 60, transdermal route of administration is preferable.

- Women with primary ovarian insufficiency may experience hot flushes, night sweats, vaginal dryness, dyspareunia, and disordered sleep.
- In women with primary ovarian insufficiency, systemic hormone therapy (HT) is an effective approach and first-line therapy to treat the symptoms of hypoestrogenism.
- Hormone therapy is indicated to reduce the risk of osteoporosis, cardiovascular disease, and urogenital atrophy and to improve the quality of life.
- Combined hormonal contraceptives prevent ovulation and pregnancy more reliably than HT.
- For a woman who prefers noncontraceptive estrogen replacement and wants highly effective contraception, insertion of a levonorgestrel intrauterine device is preferable to oral progestin therapy.

POI patients should maintain a healthy lifestyle, balanced diet, physical activity, and good sleeping habits and avoid smoking. Continuation of therapy thereafter should be based on discussion with the patient in the light of current evidence regarding risks and benefits in women taking

It should, therefore, be a public health priority that healthcare professionals are given adequate education and resources to identify the women at risk at an early stage.

References

1. Fontana L, Kennedy BK, Longo VD, et al. Medical research: treat ageing. Nature. 2014;511:405–7. https://doi.org/10.1038/511405a.
2. Albright F, Smith PH, Fraser R. A syndrome characterized by primary ovarian insufficiency and decreased stature: report of 11 cases with a digression on hormonal control of axillary and pubic hair. Am J Med Sci. 1942;204:625–48.
3. Vujovic S, Brincat M, Erel T, et al. EMAS position statement: managing women with premature ovarian failure. Maturitas. 2010;67:91–3.
4. Nelson LM, Covington SN, Rebar RW. An update: spontaneous premature ovarian insufficiency is non early menopause. Fertil Steril. 2005;83:1327–32.
5. ESHRE guideline: management of women with premature ovarian insufficiency. Hum Reprod Embriol. 2016;5:926–37.
6. Vujovic S. Aetiology of premature ovarian failure. Menopause Int. 2009;15:72–5.
7. Coulam CB, Adamson SC, Annegers JF. Incidence of premature ovarian failure. Obstet Gynecol. 1986;67:604–6.
8. Luborsky JL, Meyer P, Sowers MF, et al. Premature menopause in a multi-ethnic population study of the menopause transition. Hum Reprod. 2003;18:199–206. https://doi.org/10.1093/humrep/deg005.
9. Golezar S, Ramezani TF, Khazaei S, et al. The global prevalence of primary ovarian insufficiency and early menopause: a meta-analysis. Climacteric. 2019;22:403–11. https://doi.org/10.1080/13697137.2019.1574738.
10. Vegetti W, Grazia Tibiletti M, et al. Inheritance in idiopathic premature ovarian failure: analysis of 71 cases. Hum Reprod. 1998;13:1796–800. https://doi.org/10.1093/humrep/13.7.1796.
11. van Kasteren YM, Hundscheid RD, Smits AP, et al. Familial idiopathic premature ovarian failure: an overrated and underestimated genetic disease? Hum Reprod. 1999;14:2455–9. https://doi.org/10.1093/humrep/14.10.2455.
12. Cintron D, Rodriguez-Gutierrez R, Serrano V, et al. Effect of estrogen replacement therapy on bone and cardiovascular outcomes in women with Turner syndrome: a systemic review and meta-analysis. Endocrine. 2017;55:366–75.
13. Qin Y, Vujovic S, et al. Ethnic specificity of the variants on the ESR1, HK3, BRSK1 genes and the 8q22.3 locus: no association with premature ovarian failure in Serbian women. Maturitas. 2014;77:64–7.
14. Dittmar M, Kahaly GJ. Polyglandular autoimmune syndromes: immunogenetics and long-term follow-up. J Clin Endocrinol Metab. 2003;88:2983–92.
15. Holroyd CR, Edwards CJ. The effects of hormone replacement therapy on autoimmune disease: rheumatoid arthritis and systemic lupus erythematosus. Climacteric. 2009;12:378–86.
16. Kirshenbaum M, Orvieto R. Premature ovarian insufficiency (POI) and autoimmunity—an update appraisal. J Assist Reprod Genet. 2019;36:2207–15.
17. Bunpei I. Current understanding of the etiology, symptomatology, and treatment options in premature ovarian insufficiency (POI). Front Endocrinol. 2021;12:626924. https://doi.org/10.3389/fendo.2021.626924.
18. Takae S, Kawamura K, Sato Y, et al. Analysis of late-onset ovarian insufficiency after ovarian surgery: retrospective study with 75 patients of post-surgical ovarian insufficiency. PLoS One. 2014;9:e98174.
19. Spears N, Lopez F, Stefansdottir A, et al. Ovarian damage from chemotherapy and current approach to its protection. Hum Reprod Update. 2019;25:673–93.
20. Nillson E, Klukovich R, Sadler-Riggleman I, et al. Environmental toxicants induced epigenetic transgenerational inheritance of ovarian pathology and granulosa cell epigenetics and transcriptome alterations: ancestral origins of polycystic ovary syndrome and premature ovarian insufficiency. Epigenetics. 2018;13:875–95.
21. Bodnar AG, Quekkette M, Frolkis M, et al. Extension of life-span by introduction of telomerase into normal human cells. Science. 1998;16:349–52.

22. Slijepcevic D, Stozinic S, Vujovic S. Stres i somatizacija. Strucna knjiga. Ur: Vlahovic Z. Beograd; 1994.
23. Huang Y, Hu C, et al. Inflamm-Aging: A new mechanism affecting premature ovarian insufficiency. J Immunol Res. 2019.
24. Said S, el-Demerdash J, Tuohy VK. Autoimmune targeting disruption of pituitary-ovarian axis causes premature ovarian insufficiency. J Immunol. 2006;3:1988–98.
25. Snowdon DA, Kane RL, Beeson WL, et al. Is early natural menopause a biologic marker of health and aging? Am J Public Health. 1989;79:709–13.
26. Honigberg MC, Zekavat SM, Aragam K, et al. Association of premature natural and surgical menopause with incident cardiovascular disease. JAMA. 2019;322(24):2411–21.
27. van der Schouw YT, van der Graaf Y, Steyerberg EW, et al. Age at menopause as a risk factor for cardiovascular mortality. Lancet. 1996;347:714–8.
28. Tao XY, Zuo AZ, Wang JQ, Tao FB. Effects of primary ovarian insufficiency and early natural menopause on mortality: a meta-analysis. Climacteric. 2016;19:27–36.
29. Rahman H, Corcoran D, Aetesam-Ur-Rahman M, et al. Diagnosis of patients with angina and non-obstructive coronary disease in the catheter laboratory. Heart. 2019;105:1536–41.
30. Van Lennep JER, Heida KV, Bots ML, Hoek A. Cardiovascular disease in women with premature ovarian insufficiency: a systematic review and meta-analysis. Eur J Prevent Cardiol. 2016;23:178–86.
31. Amagai Y, Ishikawa S, Gotoh T, et al. Age at menopause and mortality in Japan. The Jichi Medical School Cohort study. J Epidemiol. 2006;16:161–8.
32. Gallagher LG, Davis LB, Ray RM, et al. Reproductive history and mortality from cardiovascular diseases among women textile workers in Shangai, China. Int J Epidemiol. 2011;40:1510–8.
33. Jacobsen BK, Knutsen SF, Fraser GE. Age at natural menopause and total mortality and mortality from ischemic heart disease: the Adventist Health Study. J Clin Epidemiol. 1999;52:303–7.
34. Wu X, Cai H, Kallianpur A. Impact of premature ovarian failure on mortality and morbidity among Chinese women. PLoS One. 2014;9:e89597.
35. Gianini A, Genazzani AR, Simoncini T. The long-term risks of premature ovarian insufficiency. In: Genazzani AR, Tarlatszis B, editors. Frontiers in gynecological endocrinology. Vol. 3. Ovarian function and reproduction—from needs to possibilities. Springer; 2016. p. 61–6.
36. Gerval MO, John S. Establishing the risk related to hormone replacement therapy and cardiovascular disease in women. Clin Pharm. 2017;5:7–24.
37. Kuylaksizoglu M, Ipeka S, Kebapcilar L, et al. Risk factors for diabetes mellitus in women with premature ovarian insufficiency. Biol Trace Elem Res. 2013;154:313–20.
38. Vega EM, Egoa MA, Mautalen CA. Influence of menopausal age on the severity of osteoporosis in women with vertebral fractures. Maturitas. 1994;19:117–24.
39. Meczekalski B, Podfigurna-Stopa A, Genazzani AR. Hypoestrogenism in young women and its influence on bone mineral density. Gynecol Endocrinol. 2010;26:625–57.
40. Lana MBP, Straminsky V, Onetoo C, et al. What is really responsible for bone loss in spontaneous premature ovaria failure? A new enigma. Gynecol Endocrinol. 2010;26:755–9.
41. Popat VB, Calis KA, Vanderhoot VH. Bone mineral density in estrogen deficient young women. J Clin Endocrinol Metab. 2006;54:2777–83.
42. Vuksanovic M, Vujovic S. Uticaj promenljivih faktora rizika za nastanak osteoporoze u zena sa prevremenom insuficijencijom ovarijuma. Beograd: Rad uze specijalizacije; 2021.
43. Luine VN. Estradiol and cognitive function: past, present, future. Horm Behav. 2014;66:602–18.
44. Rocca WA, Grossardt BR, Shuster LT, Stewart EA. Hysterectomy, oophorectomy, estrogen, and the risk of dementia. Neurodegener Dis. 2012;10:175–8. https://doi.org/10.1159/000334764.
45. Pacello PC, Yelc PA, Rabelo C. Dyspareunia and lubrication in premature ovarian failure using hormone therapy and vaginal health. Clin Endocrinol. 2014;17:342–7.
46. Nappi RE, Cucinella L, Martini E, et al. Sexuality in premature ovarian insufficiency. Climacteric. 2019;22:289–95.
47. DeAlmeida DM, Benetti-Pinto CL, Makuch MY. Sexual function of women with premature ovarian failure. Menopause. 2011;18:262–6.

48. Van Kesteren YM, Schoemaher J. Premature ovarian failure: a systematic review on therapeutic interventions to restoring ovarian function and achieve pregnancy. Hum Reprod Update. 1999;5:483–92.
49. Letru-Kornish H, Delaian S. Successful pregnancy after combined pentoxifylline-tocopherol treatment in women with premature ovarian failure. Fertil Steril. 2003;79:439–41.
50. Vujovic S, Ivovic M, Tancic Gajic M, Genazzani AR, et al. Endometrium receptivity in premature ovarian insufficiency—how to improve fertility rate and predict diseases? Gynecol Endocrinol. 2018;12:1011–5.
51. Hubayler ZR, Popat V, Vanderhoof VH, et al. A prospective evaluation of antral follicle function in women with 46,XX spontaneous premature ovarian insufficiency. Fertil Steril. 2010;94:1769–74.
52. Vujovic S, GREM. https://doi.org/10.53260-GREM.2120110. 2021.
53. Uysal S, Zekilsik A, Eris S, et al. Correlation of endometrial glycodelin expression and pregnancy outcome in cases with polycystic ovary syndrome treated with clomiphene citrate plus metformin: a controlled study. Obstet Gynecol Int. 2015;8:12–6.
54. Mamas L, Mamas E. Premature ovarian failure and dehydroepiandrosterone. Fertil Steril. 2009;91:644–6.
55. Jadoul P, Dolmans M, Donnez J. Fertility preservations in girls during childhood: is it feasible, efficient and safe and to whom should it be proposed? Hum Reprod Update. 2010;16:617–30.
56. Dragojevic Dikic S. Premature ovarian insufficiency—current hormonal approach in optimizing fertility rate—the role of melatonin. In: 18th world congress of Gynecological endocrinology. Florence; 2018.
57. NICE Guideline [NG23]: menopause diagnosis and management. https://www.nice.org.uk/guidance/ng23. Last accessed 2020.
58. Huhtaniemi I, Alevizaki M. Gonadotrophin resistance. Best Pract Res Clin Endocrinol Metab. 2006;20:561–76.
59. Barriga PP, Montel CG. POI in adolescence:an update. Gynecol Reprod Endocrinol Metab. 2021;2:2–11.
60. Panay N, Anderson RA, Nappi RE, Vincent AJ, Vujovic S, Webber L. Premature ovarian insufficiency: an International menopause society white paper. Climacteric. 2020;23:1–67.
61. Baber R, Pannay N, Fenton A, International Menopause Society Writing Group. IMS recommendations in women's midlife health and hormone replacement therapy. Climacteric. 2016;2:109–50.
62. Chiu T, Rogers MS, Law E, et al. Follicular fluid concentrations of myo-inositol in patients undergoing IVF: relationship with oocyte quality. Hum Reprod. 2002;17(6):1591–6.
63. Canpolat U. The association of premature ovarian insufficiency with ventricular repolarization dynamics by QT dynamicity. Europace. 2013;15:1657–63.
64. Daan NMP. Cardiovascular risk in women with premature ovarian failure compared to premenopausal women at middle age. J Clin Endocinol Metab. 2016;101:3306–15.
65. Goldmeier S, Angelis K, Casali KR, et al. Cardiovascular dysfunction in premature ovarian failure. Am J Transl Res. 2014;6:91–101.
66. Sullivan SP, Sarrel PM, Nelson LM. Hormone replacement therapy in young women with premature ovarian insufficiency and early menopause. Fertil Steril. 2016;100:1588–99.
67. Pearce EL. Enhance CD-8 T-cell memory by modulating fatty acid metabolism. Nature. 2009;460:103–7.
68. Pernicova I, Korbonis M. Metformin—mode of action and clinical implications for Diabetes and cancer. Nat Rev Endocrinol. 2014;10:577–86.
69. Marina LJ, Ivovic M, Vujovic S, et al. Luteinizing hormone and insulin resistance in menopausal patients with adrenal incidentalomas. The cause-effect relationship? Clin Endocrinol. 2018;4:541–8.
70. Drake MT, Clarke BL, Khosla S. Bisphosphonates: mechanism of action and role in clinical practice. Mayo Clin Proc. 2008;83:1032–45.
71. Bove R, Secor E, Chibnik LB. Age at surgical menopause influences cognitive decline and Alzheimer pathology in older women. Neurology. 2014;82:222–9.

72. Janse F, Tamahatoe SJ, Eijkemans MJ, Fauser BC. Testosterone concentrations, using different assays, in different types of ovarian insufficiency: a systemic review and meta-analysis. Hum Reprod Update. 2012;18:405–19.

73. Wong QHY, Yeung TWY, Yung SSF, et al. The effects of 12 month dehydroepiandrosterone supplementation on the menstrual pattern, ovarian reserve and safety profiles in women with premature ovarian insufficiency. J Assist Reprod Genet. 2018;35:857–62.

74. Davis SR, Baber R, Panay N, et al. Global consensus position statements on the use of testosterone therapy for women. Climacteric. 2019;22:429–34.

75. Tartagni M, Cicinelli E, De Pergola G, et al. Effects of pretreatment with estrogens on ovarian stimulation with gonadotropins in women with premature ovarian failure: a randomized, placebo-controlled trial. Fertil Steril. 2007;87:858–61.

76. Dragojevic Dikic S, Vasiljevic M, Jovanovic A, Vujovic S. Premature ovarian insufficiency—novel hormonal approach in optimizing fertility. Gynecol Endocrinol. 2020;36:162–5.

77. Ljubić A, Božanović T, Pirkovic-Cabarkapa A, et al. Live birth after an autologous platelet-rich plasma ovarian in vitro activation and bone marrow stem cells transplantation in a premature ovarian failure case report. Res Square. 2021:1–14. https://doi.org/10.21203/rs.3.rs-173188/v1.

78. Rosario R, Anderson RA. Novel approaches to fertility restoration in women with premature ovarian insufficiency. Climacteric. 2021;24(5):491–7. https://doi.org/10.1080/13697137.2020.1856806.

79. Sadeghi MR. Access to infertility services in middle east. J Reprod Infertil. 2015;16:179.

80. Liu T, Huang Y, Chen C. Transplantation of human menstrual blood stem cells to premature ovarian failure in mouse model. Stem Cells Dev. 2014;23:1548.

81. Benneti-Pinto CL, Brancalion MF, Assis LH, et al. Mammographic breast density in women with premature ovarian failure: a prospective analysis. Menopause. 2014;21:933–7.

82. Collaborative Group on Hormonal Factors and Breast Cancer. Type and timing of menopausal hormone therapy risk: individual participants meta-analysis of the world-wide epidemiological evidence. Lancet. 2019;394:1159–68.

83. Malone KE, Daling JR, Weiss NS. Oral contraceptives in relation to breast cancer. Epidemiol Rev. 1993;15:80–97.

84. Bosze P, Toth A, Toroko M. Hormone replacement and the risk of breast cancer in Turner's syndrome. N Engl J Med. 2006;355:2599–600.

85. Gordhandas S, Norquist BM, Pennington KP, et al. Hormone replacement therapy after risk reducing salpingo-oophorectomy in patients with BRCA 1 and 2 mutations: a systemic review of risks and benefits. Gynecol Oncol. 2019;153:192–200.

86. Carroll JS. Mechanisms of oestrogen receptor (ER) gene regulation in breast cancer. Eur J Endocrinol. 2016;175:R41–9.

87. Vinogradova Y, Coupland C, Hippisley-Cox J. Use of hormone replacement therapy and risk of venous thromboembolism: nested case-control studies using the Q research and CRPRD databases. BMJ. 2019;364:k4892.

88. Dunselman GA, Vermeulen N, Becker C, et al. ESHRE guideline: management of women with endometriosis. Hum Reprod. 2014;29:400.

89. Ciarmela P, Ciavattini A, Giannubilo S, et al. Management of leiomyomas in perimenopausal women. Maturitas. 2014;78:168–73.

90. Vujovic S, Ivovic M, Tancic Gajic M, et al. Chapter 5: Premature ovarian insufficiency: optimizing quality of life and long term effects. In: Frontiers in gynecological endocrinology. 2020. p. 38–47.

Menopause Is a Natural Condition: Does It Require to Be Corrected? For Whom and for How Long?

12

Tiziana Fidecicchi, Marisa Ardito, Andrea Giannini, Tommaso Simoncini, and Andrea R. Genazzani

12.1 Signs and Symptoms of Menopause

Menopause generally occurs at around 51 years of age, with an age range varying between 40 and 60 years. The World Health Organization (WHO) defines *menopause* as the permanent cessation of menses due to the loss of ovarian follicular activity.

The three stages of perimenopause set by "Stages of Reproductive Aging Workshop" (STRAW) are:

- Early menopausal transition (early perimenopause), distinguished by an irregular cycle
- Late menopausal transition or late perimenopause, distinguished by an interval of amenorrhea ≥60 days in the previous 12 months
- Early postmenopause, the first year following the final menstrual period (FMP) [1]

Midlife and menopausal transition are often perceived as a period of crisis because menopause's symptoms can be very distressing.

This condition added to the perception that declining mental and physical status might cause indirect health problems [2] and affect women's personal, social, and work lives. However, many women live this period without adverse implications [3] and perceive menopause as a natural stage of life.

Worst menopausal symptoms arise during the perimenopause phase: vasomotor symptoms, sleep disorders, and depression. Long-term manifestations of substantial estrogen decline are urogenital atrophy, skin aging, osteoporosis, and

T. Fidecicchi · M. Ardito · A. Giannini · T. Simoncini
Division of Obstetrics and Gynecology, Department of Experimental and Clinical Medicine,
University of Pisa, Pisa, Italy
e-mail: andrea.giannini@unipi.it; tommaso.simoncini@unipi.it

A. R. Genazzani (✉)
International Society of Gynecological Endocrinology, Pisa, Italy

© International Society of Gynecological Endocrinology 2023
A. R. Genazzani et al. (eds.), *Amenorrhea*, ISGE Series,
https://doi.org/10.1007/978-3-031-22378-5_12

sarcopenia, which might develop during the postmenopausal period. Vasomotor symptoms affect approximately 75% of women; they complain of hot flashes and sweating, which can be very stressful [4]. Hot flashes usually begin 2 years before the FMP and continue for 4 years after the FMP in approximately half of the women [5].

40–60% of menopausal women complain of sleep problems, particularly nocturnal awakenings [6, 7]. Insomnia, the leading sleep disorder, can be a primary disorder related to vasomotor symptoms, mood upsets, and psychosocial aspects. It can also underlie other sleep disturbances, such as obstructive sleep apnea or restless leg syndrome [8].

Loss of ovarian function causes a redistribution of body fat denoted by the accumulation of primarily visceral at the trunk, and one of the major complaints from women is increased weight [9, 10].

There is evidence that in obese women going through menopause, weight loss may reduce hot flashes, cardiovascular disease (CVD) risk, diabetes, urinary incontinence, and dementia [11, 12]. Visceral adipose tissue is an independent cause of CVD [13]. In women after menopause, the risk of cardiovascular adverse events increases [14, 15].

Indeed, estrogens mediate several functions in the vascular district to slow down the initiation and progression of atherosclerosis; they also improve vascular function, maintain and repair endothelium, and have antioxidant and anti-inflammatory properties. However, the considerably reduced exposure to these hormones during menopause might hurt endothelial cell growth [16].

Genitourinary syndrome of menopause (GSM) typically manifests 4–5 years after menopause. It includes vaginal dryness, dyspareunia, vulvar itching and burning, dryness, loss of lubrication, and entry dyspareunia. These symptoms can cause loss of libido and sexual decay. A change in sexual desire characterizes the menopausal transition, and it is reported that at this stage of a woman's life decrease in sexual desire does not depend on age. However, it is more complained between 20 months before and 1 year after the FMP [17–19].

Urinary symptoms comprise recurrent urinary tract infections, dysuria, incontinence, and voiding issues [20]. Many studies have proved that menopausal transition per se is not a determinant of urinary incontinence; the risk increases with obesity and parity, whereas the risk of urge urinary incontinence advances with age [21].

One of the significant health issues caused by menopause is the loss of bone density, which can cause osteoporotic fractures when symptomatic. This change seems to occur mainly from late perimenopause and remain silent early. Osteoporosis, a postmenopausal disturbance, is a degenerative disorder that weakens bones. It is characterized by reduced bone mineral density (BMD) and modified bone structure; the cortex becomes thin and porous, and trabeculae lose their connective structure. All these changes increase the risk of fractures [22]. The rapid bone loss starts in the first 3–5 years after menopause and mainly involves trabecular bone tissue. It involves cortical bone in 10–20 years [22].

Many studies have shown that women suffering from perimenopausal symptoms might develop other health issues in the postmenopausal period. For example, vasomotor symptoms like hot flashes might develop a higher cardiovascular risk. Indeed, women who suffered from frequent hot flashes, as compared to women who did not report this symptom, were found to have a higher carotid intima-media thickness [23].

Women with vasomotor symptoms and endothelial dysfunction during early postmenopause might be more likely to develop hypertension at late postmenopause [24]. In addition, the link between vasomotor symptoms and a procoagulant hemostatic profile has also been highlighted, and this might improve the risk of venous or arterial thrombosis [25].

Also, sleep disturbances might increase cardiovascular risk. Indeed, they have been associated with a more significant degree of calcification in the aorta and increased carotid atherosclerosis in midlife women [26, 27].

Finally, bone tissue degenerates more in menopausal women with vasomotor symptoms who have a lower spine and femoral neck BMD, and menopausal women with vasomotor symptoms have an increased risk of hip fractures [28].

12.2   When to Start Menopause Hormone Therapy?

Nowadays, the postmenopausal period includes a third of a woman's lifetime, considering the life expectancy of women in developed nations. The reducing sex steroid hormones is a critical consequence of normal aging and loss in gonadal function, and it could affect hormone-responsive tissues, including bone, cardiovascular system, and the brain. So how could women pass through this life phase? The key for living better and longer should be slowing the aging process down: the best and tailored management of menopausal symptoms is required for improving health and quality of life.

Estrogen withdrawal is the primary pathophysiological mechanism that explains the symptoms of menopause. That is why various estrogenic formulations are prescribed as hormonal treatment, which remains the best therapeutic option. Progesterone is used with estrogens in combined therapy in non-hysterectomized women to protect against the consequences of systemic therapy with just estrogen [29]. The rationale is to treat symptomatic women [30].

Absolute contraindications to menopausal hormone therapy (MHT) are estrogen-sensitive diseases (like breast or endometrial hyperplasia and cancer), severe active disease of the liver, coronary diseases, stroke, dementia, personal history, or inherited high risk of a thromboembolic condition, hypertriglyceridemia [31].

Most women with moderate-to-severe symptoms and a negative impact on quality of life must consider MHT [32]. Women with mild symptoms generally do not ask for hormone therapy. Vasomotor symptoms are the most common indication for the use of postmenopausal estrogen therapy [4].

MHT can also be useful when sleep disorders are related to nocturnal hot flashes, anxiety, or depression [33] or GSM, which negatively impacts women's quality of life and relational skills [17, 34, 35]. If vulvovaginal atrophy is the only symptom, low-dose vaginal rather than systemic estrogens are the most suitable therapeutic choice. Moreover, low-dose vaginal estrogens can improve sexual function and treat GSM symptoms, which is why they are often associated with systemic hormonal therapies in patients who also suffer from vasomotor symptoms. In this case, vaginal estrogen may be continued indefinitely [34].

If the woman has no contraindications to therapy and is not symptomatic, MHT may also be applied to prevent osteoporosis. If the effect of MHT is mainly preventive in perimenopausal years, it is necessary for bone maintenance in postmenopausal years. However, this preventive effect is probably attenuated if the therapy is started after 60 years of age [36].

The age when to start MHT is a critical factor. Scientific evidence shows that the ratio of benefits and risks for MHT is most advantageous within the first 10 years of menopause. When started during this "window of opportunity," MHT has long-term protective effects. Systemic MHT is considered a safe option for healthy women. It is advised for the symptomatic ones under the age of 60, or in any case within 10 years from the onset of menopause, after excluding contraindications. It has been proved that starting MHT is advantageous for cardiovascular risk in healthy early menopausal women but not in older women with different CVD risk factors [37, 38]. The beneficial vascular effects of estrogen are lost at later phases of more complex atherosclerosis, and this may lead to plaque rupture and thrombosis [39].

In the ELITE study (Early versus Late Intervention Trial), MHT based on estradiol resulted in a relatively slower advance of carotid artery intima-media thickness than placebo, but exclusively in women who started MHT less than 6 years after menopause [38]. This evidence indicates that MHT stops atherosclerosis and CVD development when initiated early after menopause, so the earlier the MHT is started, the smaller the cardiac mortality risk is. This rationale is relevant since atherosclerotic changes start to develop already in premenopausal age; thus, the findings align with the "window of opportunity" theory.

It is crucial to start treating healthy early menopausal women (<6 aa) to address the emerging symptoms of menopause immediately. These women may require a medium starting dose of oral (from 0.625 mg/day to 1–2 mg/day of conjugated equine estrogen—CEE) or transdermal estrogens (patch with 50 mg/day of estradiol—E2; gel with 1–2 mg/day E2) combined with applicable doses of progestogens in a sequential or continuous regimen for endometrial protection [31].

12.3 Benefits and Risks of Hormone Therapy

MHT effects on female organisms have been widely studied over the years. The therapy can positively or negatively affect different systems, which should drive the choice towards the best option.

12.3.1   Cardiovascular System and Metabolism

The relationship between MHT and CVD risk is complex. It depends on individual health status, chronological and menopausal age, route of delivery of estrogens, and dose and type of progestogen used.

It is commonly accepted that MHTs with estrogen alone or combined with progestogens are not associated with cardiovascular complications in women with a short time between menopause and the starting of MHT, independently from the chronological age. In the Women's Health Initiative (WHI) clinical trial, the hazard ratio (HR) for coronary heart disease was 0.76 in women with less than 10 years since menopause (YSM), 1.10 for women with 10 to less than 20 YSM, and 1.28 for women with more than 20 YSM [40]. More difficult is to define whether MHT could be protective against CVD risk. Some long-term studies showed that healthy postmenopausal women who started MHT early after menopause had better outcomes for myocardial infarction, death, and heart failure [41, 42]. On the contrary, older women starting MHT may already have CVD risk factors that can worsen with the therapy [43]. So, as previously defined, it is essential to evaluate the time since menopause onset when prescribing an MHT. This comprises the definition of "window of opportunity" that we previously described.

Lower risk of CVD may be obtained by administering estrogens by a transdermal or vaginal route, maybe because they affect less liver-derived coagulation factors. Even when combined with progestins, transdermal estrogen therapy is associated with a lower risk of stroke, myocardial infarction, deep venous thrombosis, and other CVD than oral estrogen-only or combined therapy [44, 45]. Vaginal E2 seems to be beneficial and safe, too [46]. The WHI observational study showed that the risks of coronary heart disease and all-cause mortality among users of vaginal estrogens were lower than those in nonusers. The incidences of stroke and thromboembolic events were similar [47].

The type of estrogen and progestogen used may affect the risk of CVD, too. Usually, CEE is associated with a higher risk than oral E2 [45]. Moreover, combinations containing medroxyprogesterone acetate (MPA) and norpregnanes (such as nomegestrol acetate and promegestone) seem to be associated with the highest venous thromboembolic risk compared to progesterone and pregnane derivatives. Norpregnane derivatives are also associated with increased stroke risk [31, 45, 48].

In general, an increased risk of coronary events while using MHT is found in women with dyslipidemia or metabolic syndrome [41, 49, 50], while healthy women can benefit from a reduction in CVD risk [51]. Also, body mass index (BMI) is important because it increases the risk of venous thromboembolism [52]. The exclusion of thrombophilic conditions is fundamental to identifying women with higher risk who may benefit from a transdermal hormone therapy [53].

Other therapies could have no impact on CVD risk. Selective estrogen receptor modulators like raloxifene and tissue-selective estrogen complex have been shown to have an excellent cardiovascular safety profile [54–56]. Little data about tibolone are available. In the LIFT study, tibolone at the oral daily dose of 1.25 mg/day caused an increase in absolute risk of stroke, and this risk rose exponentially with age [57]. On the contrary, the risk of venous thromboembolic events and of coronary heart diseases is not affected by tibolone [54, 57].

Androgens, both with the transdermal and vaginal route of administration, did not cause any serious adverse event, and they showed to be neutral on lipid profile, carbohydrate metabolism, and renal and liver function [58, 59].

12.3.2 Central Nervous System

E2 has beneficial effects on the brain, and the drop in estrogen levels after menopause can impact brain functionality. On the contrary, clinical data have been equivocal and controversial as to the benefits of MHT in the brain of postmenopausal women.

There is no doubt that MHT with estrogen alone or combined with progestogen is the best treatment option to alleviate vasomotor symptoms when low doses of estrogen are used. With the improvement of hot flushes, sleep quality also usually improves [60], particularly when natural progesterone is used [61, 62]. More difficult is to define the effects on cognition and mood.

Women using MHT, particularly those undergoing surgical menopause, usually perform better than nonusers on cognitive skills. However, the possible beneficial effects may be evident in women starting MHT early after menopause, while those starting therapy a long time after menopause usually claim worse cognitive function. As for CVD, the first studies suggested that also for brain function, there may be a "window of opportunity" to benefit all the positive effects of MHT [31, 63, 64].

More recent randomized clinical trials have shown contrasting results. Some studies have shown that MHT negatively affected cognition in women starting treatment early after menopause [65–67]. A recent analysis, on the contrary, found that the most significant benefits of estrogen or estrogen-progestogen therapy were obtained starting treatment within 5 years of menopause and that, when initiated later, MHT still produced beneficial effects compared to never users. In this study, MHT proved to be protective against Alzheimer's disease [68]. However, the relationship between MHT use and Alzheimer's disease remains to be confirmed.

As for mood, some studies tried to clarify whether E2 supplements may be beneficial or not against depression. The KEEPS trial showed that CEE associated with cyclic progesterone improved depressive symptoms compared to placebo [66]. Recently, promising results emerged also for transdermal E2 [69]. The progestin component of MHT, its dose, and route of administration may influence this antidepressant effect of E2 [31].

Regarding androgen compounds, dehydroepiandrosterone (DHEA) supplementation can generally improve cognitive function, mood, memory, and feeling of well-being thanks to the stimulation of the synthesis of neuroactive steroids and neuropeptides (i.e., β-endorphin) [70].

12.3.3   Bone

Estrogen and estrogen-progestogen combinations can prevent all fractures [36, 71–74] and increase BMD [41, 75]. MHT is the only therapy available with proven effects on fracture reduction in patients without osteoporosis in early postmenopausal years [76].

Effects on bone have also been studied with other postmenopausal therapies. For example, raloxifene and bazedoxifene are agonists of the estrogen receptor in the bone, but their efficacy in reducing fracture incidence is lower, particularly for hip fractures. On the other hand, at low doses, tibolone can increase BMD and reduce fracture risk, too; its effect is comparable to classic MHT [31].

12.3.4   Cancer

It is difficult to define a causal link between MHT and breast cancer. In the WHI study, a slightly increased risk of breast cancer emerged in women treated with CEE and progestogen, and a reduced risk was found in those treated with CEE alone [74]. In general, many authors report an increased risk after MHT, which results in higher risk mainly in long-term users. However, this negative effect has not been registered in women younger than 50 years, reassuring all those with primary ovarian insufficiency [31, 77, 78]. Vaginal estrogens do not increase breast cancer incidence [47].

It is essential to underline that estrogens and progestogens are not cancerogenic compounds. Instead, the increased breast cancer risk and more advanced cancers may result from exogenous hormones and a different hormonal balance on existing tumors. For this reason, appropriate follow-up during MHT should always be done [31].

As for women with breast cancer gene (BRCA) 1/2 mutation, who often undergo prophylactic bilateral salpingo-ovariectomy in premenopause, the use of MHT, particularly the estrogen-only MHT, is associated with a neutral or reduced risk of breast cancer. If progestogens are needed, intermittent progestin withdrawal or progestin-containing intrauterine device may be used [79, 80].

Studies on ovarian and endometrial cancer risk are consistent but not wholly conclusive. Endometrial cancer risk can be increased using estrogen-only therapies in women with a uterus [31]. Ovarian cancer incidence seems to be slightly increased in current users, particularly the serous and endometroid subtypes. This risk tends to diminish after discontinuation in a time-dependent manner [81].

12.4   Tailoring Treatment According to Age and Risk Factors

The first step approaching a menopausal woman is to create a benefit-risk profile to choose the best treatment option. Chronological and menopausal age, cardiovascular status, BMI, and breast cancer risk must be evaluated. Absolute contraindications must be excluded. Migraine with or without aura may worsen during MHT, and the lowest doses of transdermal estrogens with continuous progestogens should be preferred [82].

Once contraindications are excluded, the phenotype of the woman must be analyzed. Genazzani et al. [31] described six types of menopausal women: healthy early or late menopausal women, early or late overweight or obese menopausal women with metabolic syndrome or hypertension, women undergoing surgical menopause, and women with premature ovarian failure.

Healthy early menopausal women can take all available MHT. Usually, the first choice is medium doses of oral or transdermal estrogens, combined with cyclical or continuous progestogen to protect the uterus. Women with dense breasts may benefit from a tissue-selective estrogen complex. The addition of oral DHEA supplementation may help attenuate some symptoms, like fatigue, depression, and reduced sexual desire [70, 83].

After 10 years from menopause or at 60 years old, healthy late menopausal women should be addressed to low-dose or ultralow-dose oral, or preferably transdermal, estrogen therapy. Tibolone can also be used. Natural progesterone in a continuous regimen should be added to protect the endometrium, if necessary. DHEA supplementation can be safely used [31].

Due to its lower impact on venous thromboembolism, overweight early postmenopausal women should be addressed to a transdermal estrogen. For the same reason, dydrogesterone or micronized progesterone should be preferred [44, 45, 84, 85]. In addition, higher doses of progestogens may assure better protection of the endometrium for women with high BMI [86]. Therefore, late overweight menopausal women should prefer low doses or ultralow doses of transdermal estrogens with or without a continuous regimen of micronized progesterone or dydrogesterone, as needed [31].

Women undergoing surgical menopause are particularly susceptible to the sudden deprivation of hormones. In combination with appropriate doses of progestogen, if needed, medium or high doses of estrogens (oral or transdermal, also according to risk factors) may be used. In addition, testosterone therapy or DHEA supplementation may be added to counteract sexual problems [70, 83, 87]. Similar treatment may be offered to women with primary ovarian insufficiency, whose goal is to reach physiological E2 circulating levels until an average age of natural menopause [88]. These patients could desire contraception, too, and oral estrogen-progestin formulations may be used in this case [89].

Topical treatments can be used without restrictions for as long as it is needed if no contraindication is present. In addition, they can be used alone or combined with systemic treatments [31].

12.5   How Long Should the Therapy Be Continued?

There is not a definitive moment when to stop MHT. The decision to continue or discontinue the therapy should be based on the evolution of the health surveillance. By now, there is not sufficient data about when to halt treatment. On the contrary, many studies suggest that women receive MHT for long periods without particular risks [90]. Annual reassessment is mandatory to evaluate if new contraindications arose and if the therapy goals are met.

MHT has a protective effect against coronary heart disease that may be relevant only after several years of treatment, while it is not significant in the first years of treatment [91]. Moreover, some studies showed that MHT causes continued bone and metabolic protection [92].

As for dementia, by now, no clinical study has satisfactorily determined the effect of age versus other causes, like estrogen decrease, on the development of this degenerative disease. The mortality rates that emerged from the 18-year follow-up of the WHI study demonstrated a reduced incidence of both Alzheimer's disease and dementia in patients treated with conjugated equine estrogen [93]. With long-term treatments, no robust data about breast and ovarian cancer risk is available.

In summary, women undergoing MHT therapy should attend regular, periodic examinations, including pelvic exams, cervical cancer testing, and mammograms. Simply discontinuing MHT at some arbitrary time may not be the best option. However, women with premature menopause usually undergo hormonal replacement therapies for decades without evident effects on their causes of death, thus confirming that there is not a precise safest timing of discontinuation [90, 94].

12.6   The Effects of Discontinuation

Annual MHT discontinuation, either immediately or tapered, was a routine clinical practice to evaluate if a woman could manage menopausal symptoms without therapy. However, the acute withdrawal of MHT effects may be deleterious for cardiovascular health. In 2015, Mikkola et al. found that particularly the first year after discontinuation was characterized by an increased risk for cardiac and stroke death. These unfavorable effects were particularly evident in women less than 60 years [95]. Estrogens have a rapid vasodilatory effect; thus, an acute estrogen withdrawal may result in vasoconstriction of arteries [96]. This may cause potentially fatal myocardial infarcts or stroke. In addition, younger women may have a higher sensitivity of heart and arteries towards estrogen, a characteristic that may have been reduced or lost in older women. This may justify the higher risk of death in recent menopausal women compared to elderly women [95]. These results justify the hypothesis that MHT should be continued until benefits outweigh the risks, and annual discontinuation may not be a safe option.

Other than cardiovascular risk, 5–10% of women may develop depressive symptoms after the discontinuation of MHT. In addition, Schmidt et al. in 2015 found that the abrupt withdrawal in E2 caused a rapid increase in depressive symptoms in women with a history of perimenopausal depression [97].

On the contrary, stopping MHT causes no rebound effect on bone and no increased fracture risk. WHI data show that the benefits of MHT on bone fracture persisted over 13 years after the discontinuation of MHT [41].

As for breast cancer, the slightly time-dependent increased risk after MHT usage may partially persist for more than 10 years after ceasing the therapy. The magnitude of the increased risk depends on the duration of previous use of MHT, with only slight excess following less than 1 year of MHT use [31].

In conclusion, MHT timing, type, and duration should be tailored to the patient to achieve good compliance and outcomes for the woman and the best balance of benefit and risk possible. Overall, hormonal preparations available today have an extremely reassuring safety profile.

References

1. Harlow SD, Gass M, Hall JE, et al. Executive summary of the stages of reproductive aging workshop + 10: addressing the unfinished agenda of staging reproductive aging. J Clin Endocrinol Metab. 2012;97:1159–68.
2. Opree SJ, Kalmijn M. Exploring causal effects of combining work and intergenerational support on depressive symptoms among middle-aged women. Ageing Soc. 2012;32:130–46.
3. Lyons AC, Griffin C. Managing menopause: a qualitative analysis of self-help literature for women at midlife. Soc Sci Med. 2003;56:1629–42.
4. Woods NF, Mitchell ES. Symptoms during the perimenopause: prevalence, severity, trajectory, and significance in women's lives. Am J Med. 2005;118:14–24.
5. Politi MC, Schleinitz MD, Col NF. Revisiting the duration of vasomotor symptoms of menopause: a meta-analysis. J Gen Intern Med. 2008;23:1507–13.
6. Joffe H, Massler A, Sharkey K. Evaluation and management of sleep disturbance during the menopause transition. Semin Reprod Med. 2010;28:404–21.
7. Polo-Kantola P. Sleep problems in midlife and beyond. Maturitas. 2011;68:224–32.
8. Joffe H, Groninger H, Soares C, et al. An open trial of mirtazapine in menopausal women with depression unresponsive to estrogen replacement therapy. J Womens Health Gend Based Med. 2001;10:999–1004.
9. Lovejoy JC, Champagne CM, de Jonge L, et al. Increased visceral fat and decreased energy expenditure during the menopausal transition. Int J Obes. 2008;32:949–58.
10. Sternfeld B. Physical activity and changes in weight and waist circumference in midlife women: findings from the study of women's health across the nation. Am J Epidemiol. 2004;160:912–22.
11. Davis KE, Neinast MD, Sun K, et al. The sexually dimorphic role of adipose and adipocyte estrogen receptors in modulating adipose tissue expansion, inflammation, and fibrosis. Mol Metab. 2013;2:227–42.
12. Karvonen-Gutierrez C, Kim C. Association of mid-life changes in body size, body composition and obesity status with the menopausal transition. Healthcare. 2016;4:42.
13. Fuh J-L, Wang S-J, Lee S-J, et al. A longitudinal study of cognition change during early menopausal transition in a rural community. Maturitas. 2006;53:447–53.
14. Pou KM, Massaro JM, Hoffmann U, et al. Visceral and subcutaneous adipose tissue volumes are cross-sectionally related to markers of inflammation and oxidative stress. Circulation. 2007;116:1234–41.
15. Lee CG, Carr MC, Murdoch SJ, et al. Adipokines, inflammation, and visceral adiposity across the menopausal transition: a prospective study. J Clin Endocrinol Metab. 2009;94:1104–10.
16. Mendelsohn ME. Mechanisms of estrogen action in the cardiovascular system. J Steroid Biochem Mol Biol. 2000;74:337–43.
17. Avis NE, Brockwell S, Randolph JF, et al. Longitudinal changes in sexual functioning as women transition through menopause. Menopause. 2009;16:442–52.
18. Nappi PRE, Cucinella L, Martella S, et al. Female sexual dysfunction (FSD): prevalence and impact on quality of life (QoL). Maturitas. 2016;94:87–91.
19. Avis NE, Colvin A, Karlamangla AS, et al. Change in sexual functioning over the menopausal transition: results from the Study of Women's Health Across the Nation. Menopause. 2017;24:379–90.
20. Portman DJ, Gass MLS. Genitourinary syndrome of menopause. Menopause. 2014;21:1063–8.

21. Bolero R, Davis SR, Urquhart DM, et al. Age-specific prevalence of, and factors associated with, different types of urinary incontinence in community-dwelling Australian women assessed with a validated questionnaire. Maturitas. 2009;62:134–9.
22. Manolagas SC, O'Brien CA, Almeida M. The role of estrogen and androgen receptors in bone health and disease. Nat Rev Endocrinol. 2013;9:699–712.
23. Thurston RC, Sutton-Tyrrell K, Everson-Rose SA, et al. Hot flashes and carotid intima-media thickness among midlife women. Menopause. 2011;18:352–8.
24. Silveira JS, Clapauch R, de Souza M d GC, et al. Hot flashes: emerging cardiovascular risk factors in recent and late postmenopause and their association with higher blood pressure. Menopause. 2016;23:846–55.
25. Matthews KA, Crawford SL, Chae CU, et al. Are changes in cardiovascular disease risk factors in midlife women due to chronological aging or to the menopausal transition? J Am Coll Cardiol. 2009;54:2366–73.
26. Matthews KA, Everson-Rose SA, Kravitz HM, et al. Do reports of sleep disturbance relate to coronary and aortic calcification in healthy middle-aged women?: study of Women's Health Across the Nation. Sleep Med. 2013;14:282–7.
27. Thurston RC, Chang Y, von Känel R, et al. Sleep characteristics and carotid atherosclerosis among midlife women. Sleep. 2017;40:zsw052.
28. Crandall CJ, Aragaki A, Cauley JA, et al. Associations of menopausal vasomotor symptoms with fracture incidence. J Clin Endocrinol Metab. 2015;100:524–34.
29. Woods DC, White YAR, Tilly JL. Purification of oogonial stem cells from adult mouse and human ovaries: an assessment of the literature and a view toward the future. Reprod Sci. 2013;20:7–15.
30. Davis SR, Lambrinoudaki I, Lumsden M, et al. Menopause. Nat Rev Dis Primers. 2015;1:15004.
31. Genazzani AR, Monteleone P, Giannini A, et al. Hormone therapy in the postmenopausal years: considering benefits and risks in clinical practice. Hum Reprod Update. 2021;27:1115–50.
32. Freeman EW, Sammel MD, Lin H, et al. Duration of menopausal hot flushes and associated risk factors. Obstet Gynecol. 2011;117:1095–104.
33. Pien GW, Sammel MD, Freeman EW, et al. Predictors of sleep quality in women in the menopausal transition. Sleep. 2008;31:991–9.
34. Parish SJ, Nappi RE, Krychman ML, et al. Impact of vulvovaginal health on postmenopausal women: a review of surveys on symptoms of vulvovaginal atrophy. Int J Womens Health. 2013;5:437.
35. Nappi RE, Palacios S, Bruyniks N, et al. The burden of vulvovaginal atrophy on women's daily living: implications on quality of life from a face-to-face real-life survey. Menopause. 2019;26:485–91.
36. Zhu L, Jiang X, Sun Y, et al. Effect of hormone therapy on the risk of bone fractures. Menopause. 2016;23:461–70.
37. Savolainen-Peltonen H, Tuomikoski P, Korhonen P, et al. Cardiac death risk in relation to the age at initiation or the progestin component of hormone therapies. J Clin Endocrinol Metab. 2016;101:2794–801.
38. Hodis HN, Mack WJ, Henderson VW, et al. Vascular effects of early versus late postmenopausal treatment with estradiol. N Engl J Med. 2016;374:1221–31.
39. Mikkola T. Estrogen replacement therapy, atherosclerosis, and vascular function. Cardiovasc Res. 2002;53:605–19.
40. Rossouw JE, Prentice RL, Manson JE, et al. Postmenopausal hormone therapy and risk of cardiovascular disease by age and years since menopause. JAMA. 2007;297:1465–77.
41. Manson JE, Chlebowski RT, Stefanick ML, et al. Menopausal hormone therapy and health outcomes during the intervention and extended poststopping phases of the women's health initiative randomized trials. JAMA. 2013;310:1353.
42. Schierbeck LL, Rejnmark L, Tofteng CL, et al. Effect of hormone replacement therapy on cardiovascular events in recently postmenopausal women: randomised trial. BMJ. 2012;345:–e6409.

43. Switch Y, Warren MP, Manson JE, et al. Effects of oral conjugated equine estrogens with or without medroxyprogesterone acetate on incident hypertension in the Women's Health Initiative hormone therapy trials. Menopause. 2018;25:753–61.
44. Simon JA, Laliberté F, Duh MS, et al. Venous thromboembolism and cardiovascular disease complications in menopausal women using transdermal versus oral estrogen therapy. Menopause. 2016;23:600–10.
45. Vinogradova Y, Coupland C, Hippisley-Cox J. Use of hormone replacement therapy and risk of venous thromboembolism: nested case-control studies using the QResearch and CPRD databases. BMJ. 2019;364:k4810.
46. Mikkola TS, Tuomikoski P, Lyytinen H, et al. Vaginal estradiol use and the risk for cardiovascular mortality. Hum Reprod. 2016;31:804–9.
47. Crandall CJ, Hovey KM, Andrews CA, et al. Breast cancer, endometrial cancer, and cardiovascular events in participants who used vaginal estrogen in the Women's Health Initiative Observational Study. Menopause. 2018;25:11–20.
48. Canonico M, Carcaillon L, Plus-Bureau G, et al. Postmenopausal hormone therapy and risk of stroke. Stroke. 2016;47:1734–41.
49. Wild RA, Wu C, Curb JD, et al. Coronary heart disease events in the Women's Health Initiative hormone trials. Menopause. 2013;20:254–60.
50. Bassuk SS, Manson JE. Menopausal hormone therapy and cardiovascular disease risk: utility of biomarkers and clinical factors for risk stratification. Clin Chem. 2014;60:68–77.
51. Bray PF, Larson JC, LaCroix AZ, et al. Usefulness of baseline lipids and C-reactive protein in women receiving menopausal hormone therapy as predictors of treatment-related coronary events. Am J Cardiol. 2008;101:1599–1605.e1.
52. Heit JA. Epidemiology of venous thromboembolism. Nat Rev Cardiol. 2015;12:464–74.
53. Cushman M, Larson JC, Rosendaal FR, et al. Biomarkers, menopausal hormone therapy and risk of venous thrombosis: the Women's Health Initiative. Res Pract Thromb Haemost. 2018;2:310–9.
54. Barrett-Connor E, Mosca L, Collins P, et al. Effects of raloxifene on cardiovascular events and breast cancer in postmenopausal women. N Engl J Med. 2006;355:125–37.
55. Collins P, Mosca L, Geiger MJ, et al. Effects of the selective estrogen receptor modulator raloxifene on coronary outcomes in the raloxifene use for the heart trial. Circulation. 2009;119:922–30.
56. Komm BS, Mirkin S, Jenkins SN. Development of conjugated estrogens/bazedoxifene, the first tissue-selective estrogen complex (TSEC) for management of menopausal hot flashes and postmenopausal bone loss. Steroids. 2014;90:71–81.
57. Cummings SR, Ettinger B, Delmas PD, et al. The effects of tibolone in older postmenopausal women. N Engl J Med. 2008;359:697–708.
58. Achilli C, Pundir J, Ramanathan P, et al. Efficacy and safety of transdermal testosterone in postmenopausal women with hypoactive sexual desire disorder: a systematic review and meta-analysis. Fertil Steril. 2017;107:475–482.e15.
59. Sauer U, Talaulikar V, Davies MC. Efficacy of intravaginal dehydroepiandrosterone (DHEA) for symptomatic women in the peri- or postmenopausal phase. Maturitas. 2018;116:79–82.
60. Cintron D, Lahr BD, Bailey KR, et al. Effects of oral versus transdermal menopausal hormone treatments on self-reported sleep domains and their association with vasomotor symptoms in recently menopausal women enrolled in the Kronos Early Estrogen Prevention Study (KEEPS). Menopause. 2018;25:145–53.
61. Montplaisir J, Lorrain J, Denesle R, et al. Sleep in menopause: differential effects of two forms of hormone replacement therapy. Menopause. 2001;8:10–6.
62. Gambacciani M, Caponi M, Cappagli B, et al. Effects of low-dose, continuous combined hormone replacement therapy on sleep in symptomatic postmenopausal women. Maturitas. 2005;50:91–7.
63. Bagger YZ, Tankò LB, Alexandersen P, et al. Early postmenopausal hormone therapy may prevent cognitive impairment later in life. Menopause. 2005;12:12–7.

64. MacLennan AH, Henderson VW, Paine BJ, et al. Hormone therapy, timing of initiation, and cognition in women aged older than 60 years: the REMEMBER pilot study. Menopause. 2006;13:28–36.
65. Espeland MA. Long-term effects on cognitive function of postmenopausal hormone therapy prescribed to women aged 50 to 55 years. JAMA Intern Med. 2013;173:1429.
66. Gleason CE, Dowling NM, Wharton W, et al. Effects of hormone therapy on cognition and mood in recently postmenopausal women: findings from the randomized, controlled KEEPS–cognitive and affective study. PLoS Med. 2015;12:e1001833.
67. Henderson VW, St. John JA, Hodis HN, et al. Cognitive effects of estradiol after menopause. Neurology. 2016;87:699–708.
68. Matyi JM, Rattinger GB, Schwartz S, et al. Lifetime estrogen exposure and cognition in late life: the Cache County Study. Menopause. 2019;26:1366–74.
69. Gordon JL, Rubinow DR, Eisenlohr-Moul TA, et al. Efficacy of transdermal estradiol and micronized progesterone in the prevention of depressive symptoms in the menopause transition. JAMA Psychiatry. 2018;75:149.
70. Genazzani ADAR, Pluchino N, Begliuomini S, et al. Long-term low-dose oral administration of dehydroepiandrosterone modulates adrenal response to adrenocorticotropic hormone in early and late postmenopausal women. Gynecol Endocrinol. 2006;22:627–35.
71. Marjoribanks J, Farquhar C, Roberts H, et al. Long-term hormone therapy for perimenopausal and postmenopausal women. Cochrane Database Syst Rev. 2017;2017:CD004143.
72. Cauley JA. Effects of estrogen plus progestin on risk of fracture and bone mineral density. The Women's Health Initiative randomized trial. JAMA. 2003;290:1729.
73. Jackson RD, LaCroix AZ, Gass M, et al. Calcium plus vitamin D supplementation and the risk of fractures. N Engl J Med. 2006;354:669–83.
74. Writing Group for the Women's Health Initiative Investigators. Risks and benefits of estrogen plus progestin in healthy postmenopausal women: principal results from the Women's health initiative randomized controlled trial. JAMA. 2002;288:321–33.
75. Miller VT. Effects of estrogen or estrogen/progestin regimens on heart disease risk factors in postmenopausal women. JAMA. 1995;273:199.
76. Bagger YZ, Tankó LB, Alexandersen P, et al. Two to three years of hormone replacement treatment in healthy women have long-term preventive effects on bone mass and osteoporotic fractures: the PERF study. Bone. 2004;34:728–35.
77. Mikkola TS, Savolainen-Peltonen H, Tuomikoski P, et al. Reduced risk of breast cancer mortality in women using postmenopausal hormone therapy: a Finnish nationwide comparative study. Menopause. 2016;23:1199–203.
78. O'Brien KM, Fei C, Sandler DP, et al. Hormone therapy and young-onset breast cancer. Am J Epidemiol. 2015;181:799–807.
79. Domchek SM, Mitchell G, Lindeman GJ, et al. Challenges to the development of new agents for molecularly defined patient subsets: lessons from BRCA1/2-associated breast cancer. J Clin Oncol. 2011;29:4224–6.
80. Kotsopoulos J, Gronwald J, Karlan BY, et al. Hormone replacement therapy after oophorectomy and breast cancer risk among BRCA1 mutation carriers. JAMA Oncol. 2018;4:1059.
81. Collaborative Group on Epidemiological Studies of Ovarian Cancer, Beral V, Gaitskell K, et al. Menopausal hormone use and ovarian cancer risk: individual participant meta-analysis of 52 epidemiological studies. Lancet. 2015;385:1835–42.
82. MacGregor EA. Migraine, menopause and hormone replacement therapy. Post Reprod Health. 2018;24:11–8.
83. Pluchino N, Ninni F, Stomati M, et al. One-year therapy with 10mg/day DHEA alone or in combination with HRT in postmenopausal women: effects on hormonal milieu. Maturitas. 2008;59:293–303.
84. Shufelt CL, Merz CNB, Prentice RL, et al. Hormone therapy dose, formulation, route of delivery, and risk of cardiovascular events in women. Menopause. 2014;21:260–6.
85. Canonico M, Oger E, Plus-Bureau G, et al. Hormone therapy and venous thromboembolism among postmenopausal women. Circulation. 2007;115:840–5.

86. Ciccone MA, Whitman SA, Conturie CL, et al. Effectiveness of progestin-based therapy for morbidly obese women with complex atypical hyperplasia. Arch Gynecol Obstet. 2019;299:801–8.

87. Davis SR, Baber R, Panay N, et al. Global consensus position statement on the use of testosterone therapy for women. J Clin Endocrinol Metab. 2019;104:4660–6.

88. Nelson LM. Primary ovarian insufficiency. N Engl J Med. 2009;360:606–14.

89. Santoro N, Teal S, Gavito C, et al. Use of a levonorgestrel-containing intrauterine system with supplemental estrogen improves symptoms in perimenopausal women. Menopause. 2015;22:1301–7.

90. Naftolin F, Friedenthal J, Nachtigall R, et al. Cardiovascular health and the menopausal woman: the role of estrogen and when to begin and end hormone treatment. F1000Res. 2019;8:1576.

91. Harman SM, Vittinghoff E, Brinton EA, et al. Timing and duration of menopausal hormone treatment may affect cardiovascular outcomes. Am J Med. 2011;124:199–205.

92. Lindsay R. Hormones and bone health in postmenopausal women. Endocrine. 2004;24:223–30.

93. Manson JE, Aragaki AK, Rossouw JE, et al. Menopausal hormone therapy and long-term all-cause and cause-specific mortality. JAMA. 2017;318:927.

94. Salpeter SR, Cheng J, Thabane L, et al. Bayesian meta-analysis of hormone therapy and mortality in younger postmenopausal women. Am J Med. 2009;122:1016–1022.e1.

95. Mikkola TS, Tuomikoski P, Lyytinen H, et al. Increased cardiovascular mortality risk in women discontinuing postmenopausal hormone therapy. J Clin Endocrinol Metab. 2015;100:4588–94.

96. Ciccone MM, Scicchitano P, Gesualdo M, et al. Systemic vascular hemodynamic changes due to 17-β-estradiol intranasal administration. J Cardiovasc Pharmacol Ther. 2013;18:354–8.

97. Schmidt PJ, Ben-Dor R, Martinez PE, et al. Effects of estradiol withdrawal on mood in women with past perimenopausal depression. JAMA Psychiatry. 2015;72:714.

Printed in the United States
by Baker & Taylor Publisher Services